Evaluating & Enhancing

Children's Phonological Systems

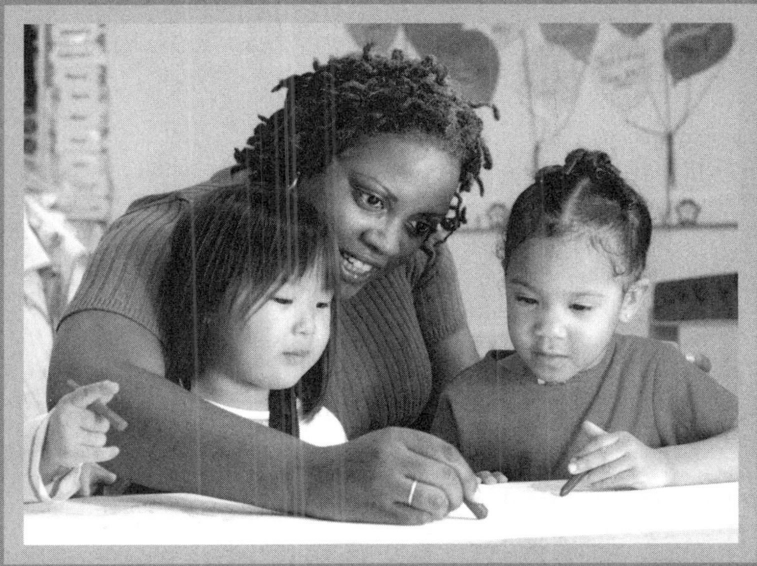

Research & Theory to Practice

Barbara Williams Hodson, PhD

Thinking Publications® • Greenville, SC

12 11 10 09 08 07 6 5 4 3 2 1

Library ofCongress Cataloging-in-Publication Data

Hodson, Barbara Williams, date
Evaluating and enhancing children's phonological systems : research and theory to practice / Barbara W. Hodson.
p. cm.
Includes bibliographical references and index.
Contents: Contents: Foundation information--phonetics and phonological acquisition--Diagnostic evaluation and treatment options--Applications for children with highly unintelligible speech--Theoretical considerations, major issues, and research needs.
ISBN 1-932054-52-9 (pbk.)
1. Speech disorders in children. 2. Language disorders in children. 3. Speech therapy. I. Title.

RJ496.S7H63 2006
618.92'855--dc22

20052056410

Printed in the United States ofAmerica
Graphic Design by Tyler Schwartz
Cover Photo ©Jupiter Images

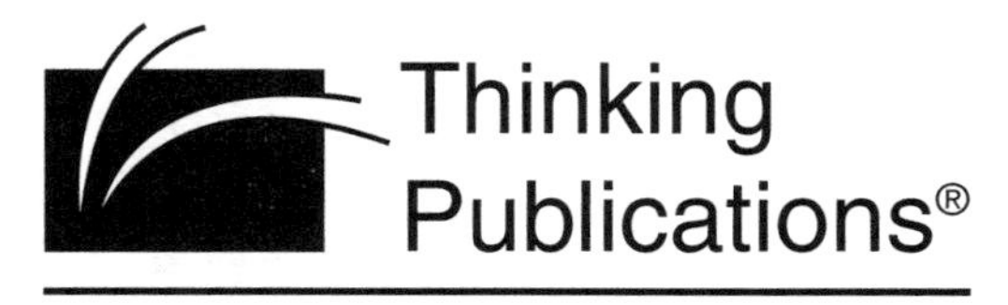

A Division of Super Duper® Inc.
P.O. Box 24997
Greenville, SC 29616
custserv@superduperinc.com
1-800-277-8737

To Kaden and Katriana Kisner,
my two magnificent grandchildren

Contents

Foreword

"Defective articulation" was one of the first two speech disorders to attract persons in the United States to devote professional careers to helping those who exhibited it. Perhaps because the inability to speak intelligibly first became a serious problem for children at the time they started formal schooling, it was their early elementary teachers who sometimes took upon themselves the task of helping these children learn how to "make sounds correctly."

It was in the early 1900s that a few women were first assigned the full-time duty of "speech correction teachers" in some of the larger city school systems in this country. It is difficult for present-day speech-language pathologists to imagine how these pioneers went about their task with no university training or even literature available for study in order to prepare themselves for the job they had assumed. The state of knowledge was so meager that virtually nothing was understood about why some children were unable to speak intelligibly, and there was literally no published or even unpublished formal research on ways to go about remediation of a child's problem. (See Paden, 1970, for more history of the profession.)

In the second decade of the 1900s, a few universities—notably Wisconsin, Pennsylvania, and Iowa—recognized that there were students on their campuses who were handicapped by being unable to speak "normally" and formally began attempting to give them assistance. In the early 1920s, a handful of institutions, including Iowa, Temple, Illinois, Mt. Holyoke, and Pennsylvania State, began to offer a course in "speech correction" (Paden, 1970). One wonders what was included and upon what information the instructors based the content of these courses.

Looking back at this bit of history reminds us that the course of development leading up to our present knowledge about and expertise in the remediation of phonological disorders has been long and slowly evolving. The early "speech correctionists" first tabulated all of the consonants that a child "couldn't make" and then proceeded to "teach" these one by one, usually as isolated sounds and in words. Choice of the sound to teach first was often based on which the child "needed most"—that is, occurred most often in his or her vocabulary. It took about half a century for our profession to absorb the realization that learning to speak intelligibly involves much more than acquiring the ability to control the articulators. I recall observing a 10-month-old child repeatedly producing a series of very adequate *r* sounds during vocal play and thinking how it could be many months before he would intentionally incorporate it into meaningful speech—indeed, that he conceivably might need to be "taught" to do so.

It was not until the early 1970s that the term phonological disorder began to appear now and then in the literature, although it took many years before there was widespread understanding in the profession about how this concept differed from an articulation problem. Indeed, there were many, both within and outside the profession, who assumed that these terms were synonyms. Most clinicians were slow to recognize how much more a child needs than motoric ability to acquire intelligible speech. Eventually, of course, professionals began to search for ways to identify what skills a child was lacking when they were difficult to understand, and how, then, to teach these skills most efficiently. Understandably, many proposals were made and tested. Chapter 9 in this book, recounting the succession of theories about how children acquire speech, and Chapter 5, reviewing major intervention approaches and methods, impress us with how broad and intense this effort has been. The review also makes clear that there is always considerable lag in the application of new knowledge to clinical activity.

The course I designed and taught at the University of Illinois in Champaign—Urbana in the early 1970s, titled "Applied Phonology," was one of the first offered in a university department of Speech Pathology (rather than Linguistics) to study child speech acquisition as more than mastering motoric skills. When Barbara Hodson undertook her PhD research, she was keenly interested in seeking methods for utilizing this knowledge clinically. We first introduced the Cycles Approach to Phonological Remediation of highly unintelligible children at the American Speech and Hearing Association (ASHA) convention in Chicago, 1977. The approach was refined and more thoroughly described in *Targeting Intelligible Speech* (Hodson & Paden, 1983; revised, 1991).

The present volume, *Evaluating & Enhancing Children's Phonological Systems,* compiled by Barbara Williams Hodson, fulfills a long-felt need, often expressed by university faculty members, for a textbook to be used in a course in phonological remediation. It wisely begins with a summary of the basics of phonetics—essential knowledge for planning and conducting efficient intervention at any level that is, unfortunately, so easily forgotten when not regularly used—and an explicit account of how a child typically proceeds in acquiring phonological skills.

Following Hodson's excellent summary of ways for diagnosing a child's phonological needs, the array of choices that are available for intervention of these needs is described at length. For further understanding of the bases of these intervention approaches, the phonological theories on which they are based can be studied in Chapter 9. Part III then focuses on the child who presents perhaps the greatest challenge to many SLPs—the one who although eager to communicate is highly unintelligible. The Cycles Approach to Phonological Remediation, which was initiated at the University of Illinois in 1975 for children with extremely unintelligible speech, is explained thoroughly in Chapter 6. A detailed illustration of the intervention for a child in this category can be perused in Chapter 7. Phonological awareness considerations for children with expressive phonological impairment are discussed in Chapter 8. In Chapter 10, frank discussion of issues, controversies, and challenges faced by our profession completes the very thorough coverage this volume makes available as a text for a course in phonological remediation.

Once again, it is notable that the development and acceptance of new revelations within our profession is a surprisingly slow process. Many individuals are just now encountering the concept of the Cycles Approach for the first time almost 30 years after it was introduced. In a broader sense, that ours is a healthy profession is revealed in that the search for knowledge and improvement in service delivery is never-ending. May this ever continue to be the case for our healthy, inquisitive profession.

—Elaine Pagel Paden

Preface

This book was originally conceptualized as an introductory text on speech sound disorders. Subsequently several new general articulation/phonology textbooks have been published. As this book evolved, it became apparent that there still was a need for a book that focused particularly on children with highly unintelligible speech, but also one that was more than a clinical handbook (Hodson & Paden, 1983, 1991) so that it could be used for college classes as well as by clinicians. *Evaluating and Enhancing Children's Phonological Systems: Research and Theory to Practice* provides the basic information that college students need to acquire and that practitioners often need to review (e.g., phonetics, phonological acquisition, overview of intervention approaches), but it has a unique focus—meeting the needs of children with severe/profound speech impairment.

Over the years our profession has served children with mild/moderate speech errors quite adequately. Our record for serving clients with highly unintelligible speech, however, has not been as good. Children with severe/profound expressive phonological impairment often have remained in speech remediation programs for years working on one phoneme at a time until a predetermined criterion for mastery had been reached.

In 1975, we initiated an experimental phonology clinic at the University of Illinois to formulate, test, and accept, reject, or modify research hypotheses. A primary finding during the last 30 some years has been that enhancing phonological patterns (e.g., /s/ clusters) (in contrast with focusing on individual phonemes such as singleton /f/ until it was mastered) has expedited intelligibility gains. We also learned that cycling patterns was more expeditious than remaining on each target pattern until it was "mastered."

Evaluating and Enhancing Children's Phonological Systems contains clinical applications as well as research results and theoretical information. Its overriding goal is to help clinicians obtain the knowledge and skills needed to serve children with highly unintelligible speech as efficaciously as possible.

Acknowledgments

First and foremost I want to thank my dear friend, Linda Schreiber, former Thinking Publications CEO and Editor in Chief, for all her efforts on behalf of this book. Not only has she contributed extensively to the final product, she also has "rescued" the book at least three times.

Next I want to recognize and express appreciation to authors who contributed chapters. Harold Edwards wrote the first draft of the chapter on phonetics and "set the tone," using questions as subheaders. After he became ill and could not finish the chapter, Julie Scherz "stepped in" and did a great job of revising and completing it. The chapters by Margot Kelman and Kathy Strattman provide a solid foundation for learning about phonological acquisition and intervention approaches. Gail Gillon's chapter on phonological awareness provides much needed information because we now know that most children with highly unintelligible speech have phonological awareness deficiencies and experience difficulties acquiring literacy. The chapter by Mary Louise Edwards on phonological theories provides both historical and "state of the art" information.

I particularly want to thank Elaine Paden for writing the Foreword and also for reviewing chapters and for her superb suggestions. Her collaboration and her generosity in sharing her expertise both in writing and in phonology have truly been appreciated.

In addition, I want to recognize and express appreciation to three other former University of Illinois professors—John O'Neill for his special support and his emphasis on the auditory system; the late Grant Fairbanks for mentoring my first research experience (while a college senior) as well as his teachings about the speech system as a servo-mechanism; and the late J. McVicker Hunt, a renowned developmental psychologist, who taught the importance of determining the learner's "match" and providing appropriate challenge accompanied by success (optimal incongruity). I also want to take this opportunity to acknowledge some special phonologists whose research, publications, and conversations over the years have contributed immensely to my knowledge base and to the clinical phonology profession—John Bernthal, Ken Bleile, Mary Louise Edwards, Gail Gillon, David Ingram, Ray Kent, Kim Oller, Larry Shriberg, Joy Stackhouse, Carol Stoel-Gammon, and Shelley Velleman.

Special recognition also go to Dale Strattman for the wonderful photos found at the beginning of each of the four parts of the book and to Tyler Schwartz for the graphic design and the great book cover. In addition, appreciation is expressed to former Thinking Publications staff members who contributed in a myriad of ways—Elysia Kotke, production manager; Lauren Margolies, production assistant, and Sara Thurs, technical editor. I also want to acknowledge the late Nancy McKinley, founder of Thinking Publications, for the invitation to write this book and for her wonderful friendship.

The clients (and their families and their student clinicians) in our experimental phonology clinics at the University of Illinois, San Diego State University, and Wichita State University deserve special commendation. We would not have been able to develop and test hypotheses and continue to make improvements to the Cycles Phonological Remediation Approach without their participation and their contributions.

Finally, the chapter authors and I want to express our appreciation to individuals who reviewed chapters and provided critiques and suggestions—Linda Carpenter, Paul Cascella, Peter Flipsen, Jr., Vicki Lord Larson, Jen McCombs, Judy Sawyer, Cori Severson, and Maggie Watson. Their comments led to extensive revisions.

Contributing Authors

Harold Edwards—Wichita State University-Kansas (Professor Emeritus)

Mary Louise Edwards—Syracuse University-New York

Gail Gillon—University of Canterbury-New Zealand

Margot Kelman—Wichita State University

Julie Scherz—Wichita State University

Kathy Strattman—Wichita State University

PART I

Foundation Information— Phonetics & Phonological Acquisition

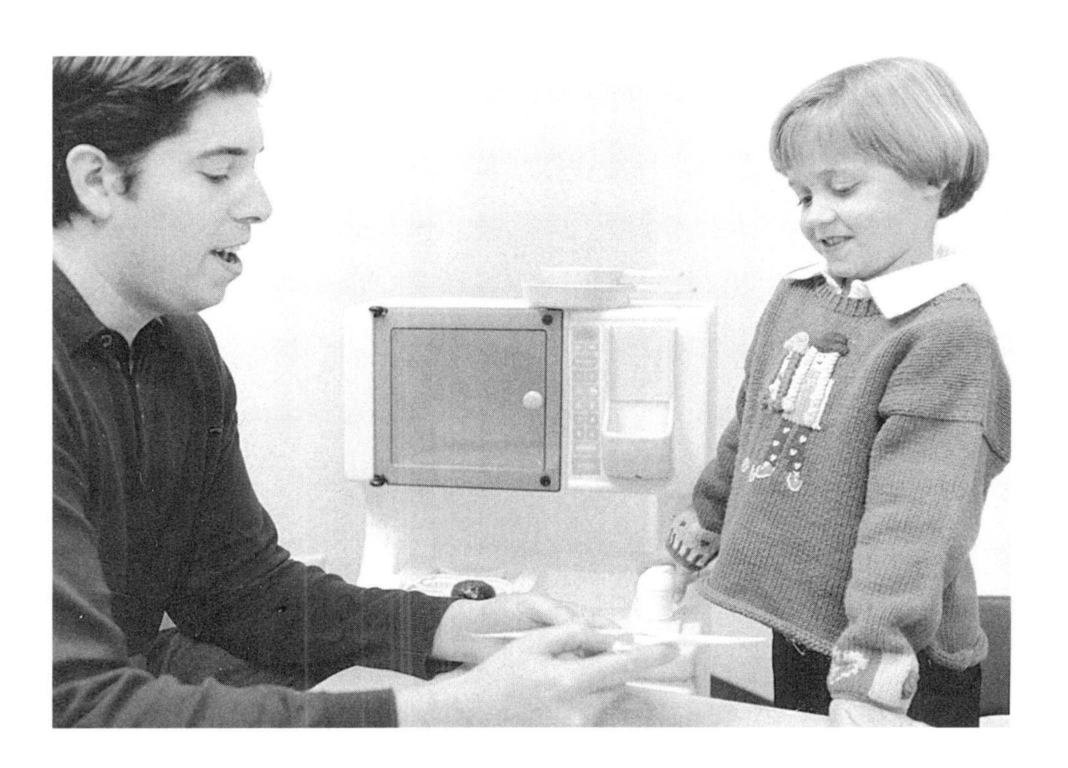

CHAPTER 1

Introduction & Overview

Barbara Williams Hodson

Purpose of Book

Importance of Expediting Intelligibility Gains

Some Basic Terms & Considerations

Overview of Book

Purpose of Book

This book has been written for individuals (from beginning students in the field of communication sciences and disorders to experienced speech-language pathologists [SLPs]) who are serving or will serve children with highly unintelligible speech. Veteran practitioners often express regret that they did not learn about phonological approaches when they were in college. Interestingly, however, many recent graduates report that although they studied various aspects of phonology in their classes, they still do not know what to do differently when planning and implementing intervention for a child with highly unintelligible speech. The goal of this book is to provide a bridge to help all clinicians better serve the unique needs of these children.

Importance of Expediting Intelligibility Gains

Two questions that often arise regarding phonological intervention are (1) Why is early identification important? and (2) Why should phonological principles be incorporated? We know that virtually all intervention practices, as well as maturation, yield gains in intelligibility. There is some urgency, however, for early identification and optimal intervention for young children with highly unintelligible speech. According to the **Critical Age Hypothesis** (Bishop & Adams, 1990), children need to speak intelligibly by age 5:6 (years:months) or literacy acquisition most likely will be hindered. This does not mean, however, that children who are intelligible by this age will not experience any difficulties; rather it suggests that children who still have major intelligibility issues at this critical age will surely have difficulty learning to read and spell. A second consideration pertains to the fact that children whose beginning reading skills are below those of their peers typically do not "catch up." Stanovich (1986) has written about this phenomenon, referring to it as **"Matthew Effects."** According to his research, the "gap" between good and poor readers widens (rather than decreases) over the years (i.e., the rich get richer and the poor get poorer).

Some Basic Terms & Considerations

Children with speech sound errors usually are assigned one of the following labels—articulation, apraxic, or phonological. **Articulation** refers to the process of producing speech sounds. Some SLPs use the term articulation to refer to mild/moderate disorders and **phoneme-oriented** tests and intervention. Childhood **apraxia/dyspraxia**—which is an extremely popular label—refers to motor planning. The descriptor currently preferred by the American Speech-Language-Hearing Association is **suspected Childhood Apraxia of Speech (sCAS)** because there are no agreed upon definitive criteria for diagnosis (see Shriberg & Campbell, 2002). **Phonology** refers to the sound system of a language. **Child phonology** involves studying: (1) **syllable/word shapes/structures** (sometimes referred to as **phonotactics);** (2) **phonemes** and **allophones;** and (3) **prosody/suprasegmentals** (intonation, rate, and stress). **Clinical phonology** focuses on identifying **phono-**

logical deviations (e.g., cluster reduction) and then determining what **phonological patterns** (e.g., consonant clusters) the child needs to learn.

It is not uncommon for a child's disorder to be called "artic," or "phonological," or "apraxic," based more on the preference of the individual using the label than on specific criteria. Some individuals use only one label for all types of speech sound disorders. Moreover, the assigned label sometimes dictates the type of intervention a child will receive. We (colleagues and clinicians involved in our clinical phonology research) prefer to say that a child with highly unintelligible speech (including a child with the label of apraxia) has an **expressive phonological impairment (EPI)** or a **disordered phonological system** and then, if the child has the potential for oral communication, to focus intervention on helping that child learn to produce and acquire phonological patterns that will result in a **reorganization** of the phonological system and ultimately improved **intelligibility.** We also prefer thinking in terms of a **continuum** (see Table 1.1), rather than an "all or none" dichotomy. The focus of this book is to help clinicians meet the needs of children in the first two categories—Profound and Severe (including children diagnosed with apraxia).

Table 1.1 *Phonological Severity Continuum for Children between the Ages of 3 and 8 Years*

Profound	*Severe*	*Moderate*	*Mild*
Extensive Omissions	Many Omissions	Some Omissions	Few Omissions
Many Substitutions	Extensive Substitutions	Some Substitutions	Few Substitutions
Assimilations Common		Distortions Common	

NOTE: Distortions and assimilations can occur at all levels, but unexpected substitutions related to assimilations are more common at Severe and Profound levels.

Adapted from *Targeting Intelligible Speech* (2nd ed.; p. 59), by B. Hodson & E. Paden, 1991, Austin, TX: Pro-Ed. © 1991 by Barbara Williams Hodson and Elaine Pagel Paden. Adapted with permission.

Overview of Book

This book is divided into four parts. Part I provides foundation information similar to that found in most articulation/phonology/speech sound disorders textbooks: Review of Phonetics (Chapter 2, by Julie Scherz and Harold Edwards) and Acquisition of Speech Sounds and Phonological Patterns (Chapter 3, by Margot Kelman). The importance of a clinician having accurate phonetic transcription skills and a thorough understanding of phonetics cannot be overemphasized. In addition, knowledge about typical phonological acquisition, including perception as well as production, is critical for the decision-making process.

Part II provides diagnostic information and also an overview of options that are available for intervention. The first part of Chapter 4 (Overview of the Diagnostic Evaluation Process for Children with Highly Unintelligible Speech) presents general information about diagnostic evaluations. The second and third parts of this chapter focus on children with highly unintelligible speech. Chapter 5 (Overview of Intervention Approaches, Methods, and Targets, by Kathy Strattman) first provides historical information about intervention approaches and programs and then includes information about the target selection process. (This chapter helps individuals understand the options and serves to prepare the reader for Chapter 6, Enhancing Children's Phonological Systems—The Cycles Remediation Approach, which focuses specifically on intervention for children with highly intelligible speech.)

Part III has a unique focus: Helping clinicians provide optimal intervention services for children with extremely disordered phonological systems. Chapter 6 presents the latest information about the Cycles Phonological Remediation Approach, which was designed specifically for children with highly unintelligible speech. Chapter 7 (Client Example—Phonological Intervention) presents the case study of a child whose speech at age 3:6 was essentially unintelligible. Initial phonological evaluation results are provided first. The goal statement and specific targets (patterns and phonemes) during four intervention cycles are provided next, followed by phonological assessment outcome measures over time (for accountability purposes). Because many of these children have poor phonological awareness skills and commonly experience reading problems (e.g., Bird, Bishop, & Freeman, 1995) and spelling difficulties (Clarke-Klein & Hodson, 1995), Chapter 8 (Phonological Awareness—Implications for Children with Expressive Phonological Impairment, by Gail Gillon) has been included. The role of speech-language pathologists in the domain of enhancing literacy has become increasingly apparent (ASHA, 2001). Moreover, recent research indicates that enhancing phonological awareness skills can have a positive impact on children's speech productions (see Gillon, 2004).

Part IV is for advanced students and practitioners. Chapter 9 (Phonological Theories, by Mary Louise Edwards) provides thorough coverage of what is currently known about phonological theories. Understanding theories distinguishes professionals from technicians, and evaluation and intervention practices must have sound theoretical bases. Chapter 10 provides a review of major issues and controversies that can affect children with highly unintelligible speech. Primary clinical research needs are also addressed. A lot more needs to be known about children with disordered phonological systems, and ultimately speech-language pathologists need to know which evaluation and intervention services are most efficacious.

Please note that in Chapters 2–8, the subheadings are written as questions. These questions can be used as study guides. The reader should be able to answer the questions after finishing the section following each question. In addition, an extensive Glossary is provided following Chapter 10 to assist the reader in understanding terms that may not be familiar. Finally, several appendixes provide additional practical information for students and practicing SLPs.

CHAPTER 2
Review of Phonetics

Julie W. Scherz & Harold T. Edwards

Introduction

The ability to speak, perhaps one of the greatest accomplishments of humans, is often taken for granted. Most of us learn to speak relatively quickly, rely on speech to meet our needs, and interpret the speech of others so easily that we rarely appreciate this amazing skill. In fact, it is only when a person loses the ability to speak or cannot speak intelligibly that the overwhelming value of speech is made evident. The purpose of this chapter is to examine speech in terms of how it is produced, which units compose it, and how those units interact.

Hundreds of languages are spoken in the world. Each uses a different number and a unique array of meaningful sounds. Essentially, American English uses about 40 **consonants** and fewer than half that many **vowels**. Some of these speech sounds are common in many other languages, some in only a few. Within a single language—for example American English—**dialects** can be found in various regions or among speakers within a particular culture or subculture that slightly alter the array and characteristics of the sounds used. Although these dialects may draw attention to themselves as "different" or "interesting," listeners rarely have difficulty understanding the persons who speak them. Moreover, we each speak a variation of our dialect known technically as an **idiolect,** an individual dialect resulting from small sound differences and voice variations that allow others to recognize us by voice alone (e.g., over the telephone).

How Is Speech Produced?

A quick review of how speech is produced may be helpful as a basis for describing the sounds of American English, the focus of this chapter. The production of speech requires that six systems work together. The respiratory system (1)—composed of the diaphragm, rib cage, lungs, and trachea—provides the power supply for speech. Speakers change the allocation of inhalation and exhalation used for quiet breathing to make nearly 90% of the air in each respiratory cycle available for speech production. Next, the phonatory system (2)—consisting of the structures of the larynx with the vocal folds approximated or adducted—serves as a valve for the airflow coming from the lungs. The air passing through the larynx becomes the sound source for speech. As the air then passes through the resonatory system (3)—either the oral cavity or the nasal cavity, the source is modified to produce different sounds. The articulatory system (4)—the lips, tongue, jaw, and palate—shape these sounds by changing the airflow in various ways. All of these systems work together in a connected sequence of events to produce the rapidly changing modifications of the airstream that produces speech sounds. This is the process of **articulation.** The nervous system (5) leads the work of the respiratory, phonatory, resonatory, and articulatory systems by directing the motor plan used by the various muscles in each system and, along with the auditory system (6), by monitoring the speech output and making adjustments when appropriate.

What Units Typically Compose Speech?

Phonetics is typically defined as the study of speech sounds, and phoneticians are the persons who study speech sounds. Some phoneticians may study the way sounds are produced by the human vocal mechanism, whereas others are interested in the product of those articulations as acoustic events. Additionally, phoneticians often study the way sounds are received by the ear and perceived by the brain. Still others examine how some sounds influence other sounds in speech or how sounds have evolved in a particular language or dialect. Speech-language pathologists (SLPs) are interested in the clinically based study of phonetics when the ability to speak intelligibly is compromised in some way. A more formal definition of phonetics is "the scientific study of speech sounds, their form (articulations), substance (acoustic properties), and perception; and the application of this study to a better understanding and improvement of linguistic expression" (Edwards, 2003, p. 2). Each of these ways of studying the sounds of speech requires its own methodology. For example, **articulatory phoneticians** require procedures for analyzing airflow, muscle potentials, and the movement of structures such as the tongue, lips, or jaw. Likewise, **acoustic phoneticians** require methods for studying sound waves.

One of the greatest contributions that the discipline of phonetics has provided is a methodology for sorting speech sounds into categories. To illustrate, consider the /ʘ/ sound, which is not used in American English. A good way to approximate this sound is to "kiss" the air, making an audible sound while doing so. The first question in the analysis might be, "Is this sound made with an accompanying vibration from the vocal folds?" The answer is "No," so it would be considered **voiceless.** Next question: "What are the lips doing during the kiss?" They are close together and rounded. We can conclude, then, that this is a **rounded bilabial** sound. Next, "What is the acoustic result of this articulatory gesture?" It resembles a quick vibration of the lips. It is a click. Therefore, the /ʘ/ sound is a **voiceless, rounded bilabial click.** To use this method of analysis on a common sound in American English, /p/ (as in the first and last sound in *pep)* is a **voiceless bilabial stop.** The /b/ sound is the **voiced** counterpart of /p/, a **voiced bilabial stop**.

Additionally, we might want to know if /ʘ/ is a speech sound used by speakers of English. We would have to locate a real word in English containing that sound. The /ʘ/ sound fails this test. It is not found in English; no words in this language include a "click." What about /p/ and /b/? Are there real words in the language containing each of these sounds? Of course, there are many, including *pat* and *bat*. The words *pat* and *bat* form a **minimal pair;** that is, they differ by only one speech sound. Further, the change in pronunciation results in a change in word meaning. Additionally, /p/ and /b/ are **cognates** (they differ only in terms of voicing). When a sound is distinctive in a language, the written symbol for that sound is set off in **virgules:** / /. When a sound is not distinctive in a language or if it is a variant of a distinctive sound, brackets are used: [ ].

Phonemes

Distinctive sounds **(phones)** in a language are known as **phonemes.** Using the criteria for describing a phoneme (e.g., the sound is found in a real word in the language, and an opposing sound exists that makes a difference in meaning), English has approximately 40 phonemes. Each language has its own set. The phonemes of English are shown in Table 2.1.

How Are Consonant Phonemes Classified?

The most obvious way to classify speech sounds is by sorting them into vowels and consonants. We add more precision to the classification of speech sounds by looking at additional ways to distinguish them from one another, namely, **manner of articulation, place of articulation,** and **voicing.** The following describes each classification system and Appendix A (see page 181) provides a Consonant Classifications Chart in summary.

Manner of Articulation

One way to classify consonant sounds is by examining what happens to the airflow through the resonatory and articulatory systems. Some consonant sounds are made with a relatively open vocal tract. These consonants are called **sonorants** and include the **nasals, liquids,** and **glides.**

The first of these are the **nasal** consonants /m/, /n/, and /ŋ/. Directing the airstream through the nasal cavity (rather than the oral cavity) makes these sounds. To do this, the **velopharyngeal port** is left open. For all other English sounds, the velopharyngeal port is typically closed by raising the soft palate

Table 2.1

Phonetic Symbols for the Phonemes of American English

Phoneme	Example	Phoneme	Example
/p/	*p*aper	/m/	*m*an
/b/	*b*at	/n/	*n*eedle
/t/	*t*ape	/ŋ/	so*ng*
/d/	*d*ate	/ə/	*a*bove
/k/	*k*ite	/ɝ/	h*er*d
/g/	*g*o	/ɚ/	herd*er*
/f/	*f*ish	/u/	h*oo*t
/v/	*v*ent	/ʊ/	h*oo*d
/θ/	*th*in	/i/	*ea*t
/ð/	*th*en	/ɪ/	*i*t
/s/	*s*ent	/eɪ/	*ei*ght
/z/	*Z*en	/ɛ/	h*ea*d
/ʃ/	*sh*irt	/æ/	h*a*d
/ʒ/	mea*s*ure	/ʌ/	h*u*t
/h/	*h*at	/oʊ/	h*oe*
/l/	*l*ight	/ɔ/	h*au*l
/w/	*w*ind	/ɑ/	h*o*t
/j/	*y*ellow	/aɪ/	h*igh*
/r/	*r*ed	/ɔɪ/	t*oy*
/ʧ/	*ch*ip	/aʊ/	h*ow*
/ʤ/	*g*yp		

Source: Edwards (2003)

(velum) to the pharyngeal wall. The second set of sonorants are the **liquid** consonants /l/ and /r/. To produce these sounds, the tongue approximates the palate, but leaves a small space through which the airstream passes. The third set of sonorants are the **glides** /w/ and /j/. During these sounds, the articulators move quickly from one position to another to modify the airstream. (As you will read later, vowels are also sonorants.)

In contrast to the open vocal tract of sonorants, most consonants are made with some type of constriction to the airflow as it travels through the articulatory system. These sounds are called **obstruents.**

The obstruents can be further subdivided. Some sounds are made with a complete occlusion (stoppage) of the airflow, which is then typically released. These are the **stop** consonants: /p/, /b/, /t/, /d/, /k/, and /g/. Other sounds are produced by various degrees of occlusion to the airflow by constricting the articulatory space and creating turbulence in the airstream. These sounds are called **fricatives:** /f/, /v/, /θ/, /ð/, /s/, /z/, /ʃ/, /ʒ/, and /h/. Finally, two sounds are produced by stopping the airstream and then releasing the air into a constricted space; these are called **affricates:** /tʃ/ and /ʤ/.

Two other terms relate to manner of articulation—sibilants and stridents. **Sibilant** sounds are produced in a way that the turbulence in the airstream causes a hissing quality. These sounds are /s/, /z/, /ʃ/, /ʒ/, /tʃ/, and /ʤ/. **Strident** refers to those sounds made when noise is produced by the turbulent airflow striking the back of the teeth. These sounds are /f/, /v/, /s/, /z/, /ʃ/, /ʒ/, /tʃ/, and /ʤ/.

Place of Articulation

Another way to classify consonant phonemes is by observing which articulators (speech structures) are used to produce them. **Bilabial** consonants are made using one or both lips: /m/, /p/, /b/, and /w/. **Dental** consonants are made by the tongue contacting the teeth: /θ/ and /ð/. These sounds are also referred to as **interdentals. Labiodental** consonants are produced by the upper teeth resting lightly on the lower lip: /f/ and /v/. For **alveolar** consonants, the tip of the tongue is placed near the alveolar ridge: /t/, /d/, /s/, /z/, /n/, /l/. **Palatal** consonants are made as some portion of the sides of the tongue touch a portion of the hard palate: /ʃ/, /ʒ/, /tʃ/, /ʤ/, /r/, and /j/. **Velar** consonants are made when the back of the tongue is placed near the **velum** (soft palate): /k/, /g/, and /ŋ/. And the **glottal** consonant, /h/, is made at the level of the partially closed vocal folds.

Voicing

A third way to classify phonemes is to consider voicing. Some consonant phonemes are produced while the vocal folds are vibrating as the airstream passes through the larynx. These are called **voiced** consonants and they include /b/, /d/, /g/, /v/, /ð/, /z/, /ʒ/, /ʤ/, /l/, /r/, /m/, /n/, /ŋ/, /w/, /j/. Other phonemes are produced without vibration of the vocal folds. These are called **voiceless** consonants: /p/, /t/, /k/, /f/, /θ/, /s/, /ʃ/, /tʃ/, and /h/.

How Are Vowel Phonemes Classified?

Vowel phonemes can be classified also. Vowels are always voiced (i.e., the vocal folds are always vibrating when vowel sounds are made). There is no constriction of the airstream as it passes through the oral cavity; thus, vowels are sonorants. The vowel that is spoken is determined largely by the position of the high point of the arched tongue within the oral cavity. These variable tongue positions cause different **resonances** (acoustic properties) to be formed. Vowels are produced according to the position of the tongue (relative to its resting position). As shown in Table 2.2, the position of the tongue can be described in terms of the distance between the tongue and the hard palate (i.e., **high, mid,** or **low),** or in terms of whether the body of the tongue is toward the front or back of the mouth (i.e., **front, central,** or **back).** Lip rounding can also influence the acoustic characteristics of certain vowels. The mid, central vowels are made with the tongue in the neutral or resting position.

Table 2.2 *Physiological Vowel Diagram*

	Front	*Central*	*Back*
High	/i/ /ɪ/		/u/ /ʊ/
Mid	/e/	/ə/ /ʌ/ /ɚ/ /ɝ/	/o/
Low	/ɛ/ /æ/		/ɔ/ /ɑ/

Source: Edwards (2003)

Diphthongs are vowel sounds that are formed by dynamic changes in tongue position during the production of the sound. When two consecutive vowel sounds are blended together to serve as a single phoneme, such as /aɪ/, a diphthong has been produced.

Vowels can also be classified by the **syllable shape.** Vowels (or sometimes syllabic consonants) serve as the **nucleus** of a syllable. Each syllable has only one vowel (or diphthong or syllabic). Consonants are added to the vowel nucleus to form various syllable shapes. Table 2.3 on page 16 presents syllable shapes for American English. For each of the syllable shapes shown, V represents the vowel nucleus and C represents a consonant.

Table 2.3 *Syllable Shapes in American English*

Syllable Shape	Example	Phonetic Transcription
VC	*up, at, in*	/ʌp/, /æt/, /ɪn/
CV	*me, too, sigh*	/mi/, /tu/, /saɪ/
CVC	*hat, top, kick*	/hæt/, /tɑp/, /kɪk/
CCVC	*skip, clap, grade*	/skɪp/, /klæp/, /greɪd/
CCVCC	*stops, preached, spent*	/stɑps/, /pritʃt/, /spɛnt/
CCCVCCC	*strengths*	/strɛŋθs/

Source: Kent (2004)

The "Unit" of Speech

What Is Coarticulation?

As speech-language pathologists, we are familiar with the English **alphabet** and the way letters—**graphemes**—are used in writing, thus it is easy to recognize that the basic unit of speech is the phoneme. While *cat,* however, is spelled c-a-t, it is pronounced /kæt/, not /k/ /æ/ /t/. Let us examine what this means.

The phoneme /k/ is the product of energy borne on air from the lungs passing through the open larynx until it is blocked at the back of the oral cavity by raising the tongue to effect a seal with the soft palate. Following a momentary pause to allow for a buildup of air pressure, the tongue moves from this position to allow the air to be released. Interestingly, this sound is actually the result of nonsound (silence), usually followed by a burst of noise. But when /æ/ is to follow /k/ immediately, as in *cat,* the vocal tract is preparing for its production while /k/ is being produced, so that the tongue is already in position for /æ/ when the /k/ is released. The two sounds are assimilating to each other. Moreover, the vowel sound /æ/, which is produced with the vocal cords vibrating and tongue shifted slightly forward and downward from its rest position, is not terminated in *cat* by simply discontinuing the airflow from the lungs as it would be if produced alone, but by abruptly cutting the air off by raising the tip of the tongue to the alveolar ridge for

/t/. Thus /æ/ and /t/ also assimilate. In connected speech, the various sounds are blended into sequences that flow smoothly together. This is the process of **coarticulation,** which subtly changes the production of each individual sound when it becomes part of a speech unit.

What Are Distinctive Features?

To understand coarticulation, it is important to examine the features of each phoneme and then determine in what contexts they might be modified. Table 2.4 shows how the phonemes in the word *cat* can be analyzed, using [+] to represent a phonetic category that is represented by a sound and [–] to show that the feature is not present.

Table 2.4 *Example of Distinctive Features for "Cat"*

/k/	/æ/	/t/
– vowel	+ vowel	– vowel
– voiced	+ voiced	– voiced
+ consonant	– consonant	+ consonant
+ back	– back	– back
– front	+ front	+ front
+ high	– high	– high
– low	+ low	– low
+ stop	– stop	+ stop

This small set of phonetic characteristics, known as **distinctive features,** helps demonstrate that we can reduce sounds to combinations of features. Turn the features on, and they result in a sound of a particular place, manner, and voice setting; turn some feature off, and a distinctively different sound occurs. For example, if the [– voiced] feature in /p/, /t/, /k/, /f/, and /s/ were changed to [+ voiced], the phonemes would become /b/, /d/, /g/, /v/, and /z/. Table 2.5 on page 18 contains a set of distinctive features for the consonants of American English.

Table 2.5 *Distinctive Features for the Consonants of American English*

Consonant Phonemes																								
	Stops/Affricates								Fricatives									Nasals/Liquids/Glides						
Feature	p	b	t	d	k	g	ʧ	ʤ	f	v	θ	ð	s	z	ʃ	ʒ	h	m	n	ŋ	l	r	w	j
Vocalic	-	-	-	-	-	-	-	-	-	-	-	-	-	-	-	-	-	-	-	-	+	+	-	-
Consonantal	+	+	+	+	+	+	+	+	+	+	+	+	+	+	+	+	+	-	-	-	-	-	-	-
Sonorant	-	-	-	-	-	-	-	-	-	-	-	-	-	-	-	-	-	+	+	+	+	+	+	+
Coronal	-	-	+	+	-	-	+	+	-	-	+	+	+	+	+	+	-	-	+	-	+	+	-	-
Anterior	+	+	+	+	-	-	-	-	+	+	+	+	+	+	-	-	-	+	+	-	+	-	-	-
High	-	-	-	-	+	+	+	+	-	-	-	-	+	+	+	+	-	-	-	+	-	-	+	+
Low	-	-	-	-	-	-	-	-	-	-	-	-	-	-	-	-	+	-	-	-	-	-	-	-
Back	-	-	-	-	+	+	-	-	-	-	-	-	-	-	-	-	-	-	-	+	-	-	+	-
Rounded	-	-	-	-	-	-	-	-	-	-	-	-	-	-	-	-	-	-	-	-	-	+	+	-
Distributed	-	-	-	-	-	-	+	+	-	-	-	-	-	-	+	+	-	-	-	-	-	-	+	+
Nasal	-	-	-	-	-	-	-	-	-	-	-	-	-	-	-	-	-	+	+	+	-	-	-	-
Lateral	-	-	-	-	-	-	-	-	-	-	-	-	-	-	-	-	-	-	-	-	+	-	-	-
Continuant	-	-	-	-	-	-	-	-	+	+	+	+	+	+	+	+	+	-	-	-	+	+	+	+
Tense	+	-	+	-	+	-	+	+	+	-	+	-	+	-	+	-	-	-	-	-	+	-	-	-
Voiced	-	+	-	+	-	+	-	+	-	+	-	+	-	+	-	+	-	+	+	+	+	+	+	+
Strident	-	-	-	-	-	-	+	+	+	+	-	-	+	+	+	+	-	-	-	-	-	-	-	-
	p	b	t	d	k	g	ʧ	ʤ	f	v	θ	ð	s	z	ʃ	ʒ	h	m	n	ŋ	l	r	w	j

Source: Chomsky & Halle (1968)

Features are powerful tools for analyzing sounds, changing sounds into other sounds, and understanding why some sounds change when they coarticulate with or assimilate to other sounds. Note what happens to the final /t/ of *bet* when placed in the word *better.* The [– voiced] feature changes to [+ voiced] when /t/ occurs between the two vowels in this context. Both vowels are voiced; thus it is more economical to leave the voice on for the /t/.

Phonetic Transcription

The symbols used by phoneticians to identify the phonemes of any spoken language are those of the alphabet designed by the **International Phonetic Association (IPA).** These symbols are illustrated in Table 2.6 on page 19. Because

Table 2.6 *The Alphabet of the International Phonetic Association*

	Bilabial	Labiodental	Dental	Alveolar	Postalveolar	Retroflex	Palatal	Velar	Uvular	Pharyngeal	Glottal
Plosive	p b			t d		ʈ ɖ	c ɟ	k ɡ	q ɢ		ʔ
Nasal	m	ɱ		n		ɳ	ɲ	ŋ	ɴ		
Trill	ʙ			r					ʀ		
Tap or Flap		ⱱ		ɾ		ɽ					
Fricative	ɸ β	f v	θ ð	s z	ʃ ʒ	ʂ ʐ	ç ʝ	x ɣ	χ ʁ	ħ ʕ	h ɦ
Lateral fricative				ɬ ɮ							
Approximant		ʋ		ɹ		ɻ	j	ɰ			
Lateral approximant				l		ɭ	ʎ	ʟ			

NOTE: When symbols appear in pairs, the one to the right represents a voiced consonant. Shaded areas denote articulations judged impossible.

Source: The International Phonetic Association (2005)

the IPA alphabet is "international;" there are more symbols in it than are needed to represent American English. The human speech mechanism is capable of producing more distinctive sounds than Americans typically use. Occasionally, SLPs encounter a child who is using a sound that would be distinctive in another language. One example is the glottal stop, in which the airstream is abruptly cut off by the vocal folds, followed by an audible voiceless release. In the phonetic alphabet, the symbol for this is /ʔ/. It is important to remember that these symbols represent phonemes, or distinctive sounds, as described earlier.

What Are Diacritics?

Using the IPA symbols, it is possible to make a permanent record of the actual way an utterance is spoken. Speaker modifications or variations may be shown by using **diacritics,** or special markings that reflect these variations. (Table 2.7 on page 20 provides a list of diacritic symbols and their uses.)

All phonemes can be made with slight variations that do not make a difference in meaning. For example, /s/ can be produced with the tongue tip elevated or lowered behind the teeth, or with the tongue tip slightly retracted. These variations in production are referred to as **allophones.** Some phoneticians would suggest that a phoneme is really a set of allophones that are all perceived in the same way. Diacritics provide a way to represent allophonic variations of various speakers and dialects.

Table 2.7 **Diacritics**

Symbol	Modification/Variation	Symbol	Modification/Variation
[̪]	Dentalization	[‿]	Connects sounds
[̃]	Nasalization, nasal release	[̝]	Raised
[ω]	Lip-rounding	[̞]	Lowered
[̥]	Devoicing of voiced sound	[˧]	Fronted
[̬]	Voicing of voiceless sound	[꜔]	Backed
[ʿ]	or [ʰ] Aspirated	[ˈ]	Primary stress
[ʾ]	or [˺] Released without heavy aspiration	[ˌ]	Secondary stress
[¯]	Not released	[/]	Short pause
[:]	Lengthened	[//]	Long pause (respiratory)

Source: Edwards (2003)

How Are IPA Alphabet Symbols Used Clinically?

Clinical applications of the use of the IPA alphabet may require modified symbols or special diacritics for capturing the precise way that a word, phrase, or sentence was uttered. For example, to explain why the /t/ in *letter* sounds more like a /d/ when the word is spoken aloud, the diacritic [̬] is placed below the /t/ as it is transcribed to indicate that it is voiced in that particular context. Clinically, diacritics can also show **distortions** (errors of precision in phoneme production).

The value of having a standard phonetic alphabet to be able to transcribe actual speech is easy to understand and the applications are many. The speech of children as they acquire their native language can be transcribed. Permanent records of dialects, some of which have only a few speakers left to provide the historical record, can be maintained. The sound system of a language may be analyzed or studied as a process of historical change, or the repertoires of various languages may be compared to determine differences or problem areas for learners of those languages. Moreover, the clinical applications are as numerous as the clients with whom we work, ranging from the speech of an individual who is deaf to others with learning, neurological, or age-related disabilities that create a myriad of phonological challenges.

The byproducts of becoming a skilled transcriber far outweigh the effort required to initially learn phonetic transcription. For example, you gain an understanding of how the sound system of a language functions. You develop an "ear" that is sensitive to different pronunciations, such as those that occur in the accented speech of those learning another language, or from individuals whose speech has been altered by accident, disease process, or age. Finally, you become a better decision-maker in the process of helping to modify the speech of others. Many resources (e.g., Edwards & Gregg, 2003; Small, 2005) are available for further review. In addition, two websites provide excellent opportunities to hear and see individual speech sounds with their corresponding phonetic symbols:

- The UCLA Phonetics Lab Archive
  http://archive.phonetics.ucla.edu/

- The University of Iowa Phonetics Animation Lab
  http://www.uiowa.edu/~acadtech/phonetics/about.html

Summary

Speech is a human behavior that is as variable as each individual. Yet, it is possible to make a permanent record of speech and its variations by using a phonetic alphabet. In addition to providing a universal alphabet, phonetics is a discipline that provides methods for studying how sounds are produced, what they sound like, how they interact with other sounds, and ultimately how the brain interprets them. From among the articulatory possibilities of the human vocal tract, a particular language selects a subset of speech sounds, the phonemes for that language. Each distinctive speech sound may be further analyzed into the features that make the sound unique within the set.

Phonetic, phonemic, and linguistic methodologies are incorporated and expanded in the phonological approach to sound classification and analysis. Once the phonemes of a language have been identified, along with their features, the phonologist considers the ways that the sounds are sequenced. For example, which consonants can occur in **prevocalic** (initial), **intervocalic** (medial), and **postvocalic** (final) positions in the syllable or word? Which sounds can occur with other sounds (i.e., can form consonant clusters; e.g., /st/ and /spl/), and which cannot (e.g., /ʒ/)? Phonology provides us with practical applications for the basic information provided by our understanding of phonetics. Much of what follows in the remaining chapters deals with phonology.

CHAPTER 3

Acquisition of Speech Sounds & Phonological Patterns

Margot E. Kelman

Speech Perception

- What Is Speech Perception?
- Are Infants "Prewired" to Perceive Speech Sound Contrasts?

Infant Speech Production

- What Are the Major Milestones of Infant Speech Development?
- What Is the Transition from Babbling to Meaningful Speech?
- What Are Vocables and Protowords and Why Are They Important?
- What Commonalities Exist in a Child's First Words?

Sound System Development

- What Can Be Learned from the Large-Scale, Cross-Sectional Studies?
- What Can Be Learned from Longitudinal Studies?
- How Can Norms Be Applied Clinically?

Patterns of Development

- What Are Patterns of Speech Sound Development?
- What Phonological Patterns/Processes Occur in Typical Development?

Individual Differences

Summary

The acquisition of speech and language skills is a monumental task. A child must gain command of several components of the language system (phonology, morphology, semantics, syntax, and pragmatics) to be a successful language user and communicator. Amazingly, most of this development takes place during the first five years of life.

Child language development can be divided into two primary periods: **prelinguistic**—which includes vocalizations prior to the first true words—and **linguistic**—which begins with the appearance of the first words. Prelinguistic skills are considered precursors to linguistic development because they lack a specific referent or communicative intent. Even so, these early skills (e.g., speech perception, infant speech production, and the transition from babbling to meaningful speech) do affect the foundation for phonological development as the first year of life lays the groundwork for speech, language, and communication.

The acquisition of speech sounds and the development of phonological skills, known as **phonological acquisition,** is a complex motor and linguistic process that begins in infancy and continues through the early school years. This process is the focus of this chapter. Speech perception, infant speech production, and the transition from babbling to meaningful speech are discussed. Phonological acquisition (sound system development) is explained from both a phoneme perspective and a universal pattern perspective. Finally, the role individual differences play in speech sound development is examined.

Speech Perception

What Is Speech Perception?

Before this chapter reviews the progression of infant speech development, a discussion about **speech perception** is relevant. Speech perception is the identification of speech sounds from auditory cues. The ability to identify and discriminate among speech sounds is essential to comprehending a language system. Remarkably, very young infants are capable of differentiating most of the sounds used in speech.

Are Infants "Prewired" to Perceive Speech Sound Contrasts?

Extensive research in the area of speech perception has been conducted since the 1970s. Two research methods—the **high-amplitude sucking technique** and the **visually reinforced head-turn method**—have been used to examine infant speech perception. The high-amplitude sucking technique tests speech perception in infants from birth to 5 months of age. The infant controls the presentation of a speech stimulus by the rate of sucking on a pacifier attached to a pressure transducer (e.g., when a new sound is introduced, an infant may acknowledge it by sucking harder on the pacifier). The visually reinforced head-turn method is a localization technique to test speech perception in infants 6 to 12 months of age. A head turn toward the sound source is anticipated when a new sound source is presented.

The high-amplitude sucking technique and the visually reinforced head-turn method are forms of operant conditioning. These studies, which are experiments in learning, demonstrate an ability to learn to respond to speech sounds and an ability to be conditioned to respond differently to different speech sounds. The experiments are not a test of innate ability in the true sense; however, they do begin to yield a picture of the infant's perceptual abilities prior to the onset of speech production.

Speech scientists have hypothesized that infants come "prewired" to perceive minimal differences in speech sounds. For example, Eimas, Siqueland, Jusczyk, and Vigorito (1971) incorporated the high-amplitude sucking technique and found that infants as young as 1 month were capable of perceiving the fine distinction in voicing between syllables [bɑ] and [pɑ]. These scientists suggested that infant perception is adult-like and linguistically relevant.

Some suggest that the young infant's capacity to discriminate speech contrasts is not limited to those that occur in the infant's immediate environment. In other words, young infants have the capacity to discriminate phonetic contrasts in any of the world's languages. Infants from English-speaking homes were able to discriminate a contrast between two sounds that occur in the Czech language, as well as a nasalized versus nonnasalized vowel distinction that occurs in Polish and French (Trehub, 1976). Two investigators who used the visually reinforced head-turn method (Eilers, 1980; Kuhl, 1987) found children as young as 2 to 3 months of age were able to discriminate place of articulation in syllable-initial [b], [d], and [g]. Evidence of discrimination of nonnative contrasts was found by Streeter (1976), who studied Kikuyu infants (in Kenya), and by Lasky, Syrdal-Lasky, & Klein (1975), who studied Guatemalan (Spanish-speaking) infants. Both groups discriminated the English [bɑ]–[pɑ] contrast even though it did not occur in the language spoken in their native environments. All of these studies provide evidence of infants having an innate or "prewired" sense of speech perception.

For a child to acquire a specific language, the infant brain must develop a structure that differentiates the child's native language from all other languages. As the infant brain takes in specific sounds and words of a particular language, it actually "prunes" neural connections that are never used (Chugani, 1994; Huttenlocher, 1994). These neural connections are reduced or condensed. Sounds that are heard frequently become strengthened and stimulated; these form the foundation for the native language (Cheour et al., 1998). This is a truly amazing process in developing speech and language skills.

Abundant research in speech perception has not pinpointed which perceptual capacities infants are born with and which they learn from the environment. Nevertheless, we do know that perceptual development is an essential precursor to speech production.

Infant Speech Production

Early theories of speech sound acquisition focused on the production of a child's first meaningful words; vocal behaviors occurring prior to the one-word stage were thought to bear no relationship to the development of meaningful speech. Further studies have shown that infant vocalizations have a direct correlation to the development of meaningful speech. All infants pass through similar stages of vocal development, regardless of their linguistic environment.

The earliest stages are influenced by the infant's vocal mechanism, which is anatomically different from that of a mature adult (see Figure 3.1). Vowel production appears to dominate infant vocalizations during the first year of life. Between 4 and 6 months of age, increased separation of the oral and nasal cavities, an alteration in the shape of the oral cavity as teeth appear, and increased tongue mobility allow the infant to produce a wider variety of sound types; that is, an expanded **phonetic repertoire** (Stoel-Gammon & Dunn, 1985).

Figure 3.1 *Comparison of Infant and Adult Oral Structures*

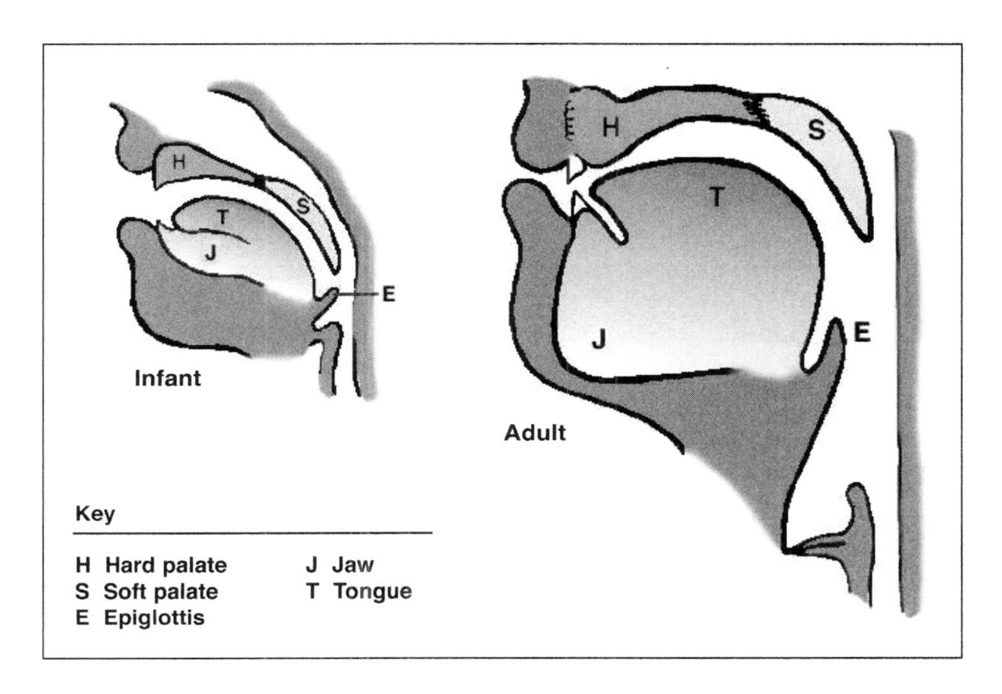

From "Acoustic Features of Infant Vocalic Utterances at 3, 6, and 9 months," by R. D. Kent and A. D. Murray, 1982, *Journal of the Acoustical Society of America, 72*, p. 353. © 1982 by the American Institute of Physics. Reprinted with permission.

What Are the Major Milestones of Infant Speech Development?

Researchers have studied and identified milestones that occur as infants acquire speech sounds. Oller (1980) and Stark (1980) compared descriptions of speech sound development over the first year of life and highlighted two key themes: (1) infant vocalizations develop in an ordered sequence of *stages* from birth to the onset of meaningful speech, and (2) the speech sounds and syllable structures characteristic of the later babbling period closely resemble the sounds and syllable structures of first words (Stoel-Gammon, 1992). Oller proposed five specific prelinguistic stages that mark the acquisition of articulation and phonological skills during the first year of speech sound acquisition. Oller's stages, summarized in Table 3.1, on page 28, are widely accepted and frequently cited in literature pertaining to prelinguistic vocalizations.

Table 3.1 *Stages of Speech Sound Development*

Stage 1: Phonation Stage (birth to 1 month)
Reflexive vocalizations (e.g., crying, fussing, coughing, sneezing, and burping) are predominate in this stage. Some nonreflexive sounds (e.g., vocalizations resembling vowels or syllabic nasals) may occur. Speech-like sounds are rare. These sounds (also called **quasi-resonant nuclei)** appear to be precursors to vowels.
Stage 2: Coo and Goo Stage (2 to 3 months)
Productions are acoustically similar to back vowels or to syllables consisting of back consonants and back vowels (e.g., CV syllables). The syllables at this stage are considered primitive because they are not well-formed, mature syllabic productions. These articulations are precursors to consonant productions.
Stage 3: Exploration-Expansion Stage (4 to 6 months)
A time of vocal play in which the child gains better control of the laryngeal and articulatory mechanisms. Productions consist of squeals, growls, yells, raspberries, friction noises, and isolated vowel-like sounds (fully resonant nuclei). These productions, termed marginal babbling, are precursors to syllable production.
Stage 4: Canonical Babbling Stage (7 to 9 months)
Vocalizations in this stage consist of consonant-vowel (CV) syllables that have more adult-like timing for closure and opening. Sounds resemble true consonants and vowels. This period is most noted for reduplicated syllables, in which sequences such as [bababa] and [mama] occur, although there is no sound-to-meaning correspondence. The infant's phonetic repertoire, although limited, may consist of stops /b, p, t, d, k, g/; nasals /m, n, ŋ/; and glides /w, j/.
Stage 5: Variegated Babbling Stage (10 to 12 months)
Productions continue as consonant-vowel (CV) sequences, but with a variety of vowels and consonants (e.g., [bawadu]). The child's consonantal repertoire increases substantially during this stage. Adult-like intonation patterns emerge.

Source: Oller (1980)

Although Oller refers to these behaviors as stages, considerable overlap occurs from one stage to another. In addition, due to individual variation, ages are given as approximates within an age range. Professionals—including speech-language pathologists and early childhood educators—and parents can refer to these stages to determine if a child is developing within typical age expectations.

What Is the Transition from Babbling to Meaningful Speech?

The transition from babbling to meaningful speech is an important milestone in the acquisition of articulation and phonological skills. The child progresses from **prelinguistic** to **linguistic** development. The most important development in this period is the linking of sound patterns with meaning, first in comprehension and then in word meaning. An "overlap" period occurs in which babbled utterances and meaningful speech are used concurrently, sometimes within a single utterance (Stoel-Gammon & Dunn, 1985). The transition from babbling to meaningful speech may last from a few weeks to several months, typically during the age period of 9 to 18 months. The transition period begins with the onset of comprehension of adult language and ends when the child is using approximately 50 different words spontaneously.

There is evidence to support three distinct conclusions regarding the factors involved in the transition from babbling to meaningful speech. First, babbling production is clearly rooted in a biological base common to all children (Kent, 1984; Locke, 1983). Second, phonetic production is shaped by the language the child is exposed to even before first words are attempted (deBoysson-Bardies, Halle, Sagart, & Durand, 1989). Third, individual children follow individual paths, drawing their lexicon from the phonetic repertoire established during the babbling period (Stoel-Gammon & Cooper, 1984; Vihman, Ferguson, & Elbert, 1986).

What Are Vocables and Protowords and Why Are They Important?

Vocables are utterances that sound like real words, but they do not qualify as true words. They are nonmeaningful. For instance, a single or repeated vowel might be considered a vocable. Vocables are not generalized, but rather, are tied to specific context and may be accompanied by a consistent gesture.

A child's first meaningful vocal productions are called **protowords** (Menn, 1975). Also known as invented words, phonetically consistent forms, and quasi-words, protowords function as real words for the infant, even though they are not based on the adult model. An example of a protoword would be production of the sound "e-e-e" whenever the infant requests a specific object. Protowords are considered the link between babbling and adult-like speech. They are often tied to a specific context and accompanied by a gesture. Because protowords do not have the stable sound-meaning relationships characteristic of adult words, however, they do not qualify as "true words." Protowords have some phonetic and semantic content; thus they usually are not considered babbling.

What Commonalities Exist in a Child's First Words?

During the period of protoword production, attempts are made to pronounce words based on the adult model; however, the child's production can be quite different from the adult version. Without assistance from linguistic and situational context, words can be challenging to identify. Common patterns can be found in a child's first words. The child begins by producing single syllables or fully or partially reduplicated syllables. The primary consonantal sounds produced during the phase of first "real" words (stops /b, p, t, d, k, g/; nasals /m, n, ŋ/; and glides /w, j/) are the same sounds that are predominant in the late babbling period.

The linguistic phase begins around the child's first birthday when the first meaningful word is typically produced. Considerable individual differences exist in the **first-word stage.** Some investigators have found that children tend to select words with sounds and syllable shapes they can produce and may avoid words with structures outside their repertoire. For example, Schwartz and Leonard (1982) presented children with nonsense words and found that imitation and spontaneous production of these words were more likely to occur if the syllabic structures and phonemes of the nonsense words were present in the child's own productions.

The linguistic phase includes the child's first 50 words. This stage extends from the time of the first meaningful utterance, beginning at about 12 months of age to the period when the child combines two "words" together at 18 to 24 months. The number 50 is merely an approximation—some children may produce fewer than 50 words before moving on to the two-word stage—others may have a vocabulary considerably larger than 50 words. As a general rule, the end of the child's first-word stage is characterized by (1) a rapid increase in vocabulary, and (2) the development of a systematic relationship between the sounds of the adult model and the child's pronunciation (Stoel-Gammon & Dunn, 1985).

Once a child enters the linguistic phase, phonological development proceeds rapidly. Phonological acquisition does not occur in isolation; rather, it develops within a language framework, influenced by cognitive, perceptual, motor, and environmental factors. These factors all have a significant role in developing the child's rule-based production system.

Sound System Development

Since the 1930s, two types of investigations have attempted to establish developmental norms for speech sound acquisition: (1) large-scale, cross-sectional studies, which are formal studies that include large numbers of participants at varying ages and (2) longitudinal studies, which follow a single child or a very small group of children over time.

What Can Be Learned from the Large-Scale, Cross-Sectional Studies?

Findings from large-scale cross-sectional studies indicate that there are universal, or near-universal, patterns of order of consonant sound acquisition (described in the paragraphs that follow). A wide range of variability exists in these studies for ages of mastery for individual sounds however. Table 3.2, on page 32, lists these studies.

Methodological differences between the studies listed in Table 3.2 are considerable. For example, they differ in when and where the studies were conducted, the size and characteristics of the samples that were used, the method and procedures that were followed, the criteria for mastery that were used, and the sound positions that were tested (Smit, 1986; Stoel-Gammon & Dunn, 1985; Vihman, 1998a). Such variability contributes to a lack of consensus in norms for individual sounds.

The criteria used to determine whether the child "mastered" a particular sound is a case in point. In Poole's (1934) study, mastery was defined as 100% correct. Two other studies (Prather, Hendrick, & Kern, 1975; Templin, 1957) used 75%

Table 3.2 *Major Cross-Sectional Production Studies in the United States*

Research Date	Authors	Number of Subjects	Age Range	Word Position[a]	Type of Production[b]	Criterion for Mastery
1931	Wellman et al.	204	2:0 – 4:0	I, M, F	Sp, Im	75%
1934	Poole	140	2:5 – 8:5	I, M, F	Sp	100%
1957	Templin	480	3:0 – 8:0	I, M, F	Sp, Im	75%
1963	Snow	438	6:5 – 8:7	I, M, F		
1967	Bricker	90	3:0 – 5:0	I	Im	
1971	Olmstead	100	1:3 – 4:6	I, M, F	Sp	
1972	Sax	535	5:0 – 10:0	I, M, F	Sp	93%
1975	Prather et al.	147	2:0 – 4:0	I, F	Sp, Im	75%
1976	Arlt, Goodban	240	3:0 – 5:6	I, M, F	Im	75%
1990	Smit et al.	997	3:0 – 9:0	I, F	Sp, Im	75%

NOTE: [a] I = Initial; M = Medial; F = Final [b] Sp = Spontaneous, Im = Imitative

From *Articulation and Phonological Disorders* (p. 106), by J. Bernthal and N. Bankson, 2004, Needham Heights, MA: Allyn & Bacon. © 2004 by Allyn & Bacon. Reprinted with permission.

correct for mastery. To complicate things further, Templin used the 75% cut-off level for all three word positions (initial, medial, and final), whereas Prather et al. used only two word positions (initial and final) in their study.

Even though there were considerable methodological differences across the studies, some generalizations can be made. On the whole, most studies found stops /b, p, t, d, k, g/; nasals /m, n, ŋ/; and glides /w, j/ to be mastered early, followed later by fricatives /f, v, θ, ð, s, z, ʃ, ʒ, h/; affricates /ʧ, ʤ/; and liquids /r, l/.

Taken one step further, Sander (1972) reanalyzed the data of Wellman, Case, Mengert, and Bradbury (1931) and Templin (1957) and developed an average age estimate and upper age limit for consonant production. Sander's data are presented in Figure 3.2. Sander's "average" criterion was based on the point at which 51% of the children produced the sound correctly in at least two positions. This **age of customary production** was compared with the age at which 90% of the children produced the sound in two positions. Sander's reinterpretation identified specific consonants that develop at the youngest age grouping, including /p, m, h, n, w,

Figure 3.2 *Sander's (1972) Consonant Acquisition*

Average age estimates and upper age range limits of customary consonant production. The solid bar corresponding to each sound starts at the median age of customary articulation; it stops at an age level at which 90% of all children are customarily producing the sound.

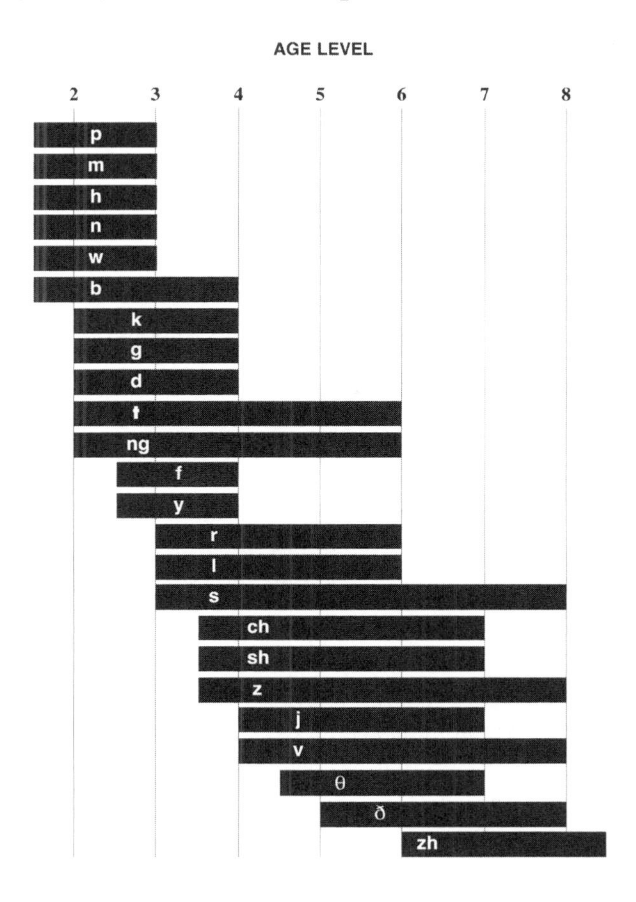

From "When Are Speech Sounds Learned?" by E. K. Sander, 1972, *Journal of Speech and Hearing Disorders, 37,* p. 62.

b/. The latest developing consonants were "th" (voiced, as in *there,* and voiceless, as in *thumb)* and "zh" (as in *measure).* Some consonants appeared to cover a wide age span, but these results can be misleading. For example, /s/ is produced correctly in some children by age 3 years; however, the upper age limit of 8 years was due to the inclusion of children with distortions of /s/ and /z/ (i.e., lisps). The consonant /t/ also has a long age span for mastery (from ages 2 to 6 years) on Sander's chart. In actuality, it should be in the early developing grouping, but the Templin data used the target word *button* and did not give credit for the glottal stop allophone, thus giving the appearance of later mastery.

What Can Be Learned from Longitudinal Studies?

Longitudinal studies revealed considerable variation in the order of acquisition of specific phonemes. For example, Macken (1980) found no consistent order for acquisition of stop consonants, and Edwards (1979a, 1979b) concluded that there was no universal order for fricative acquisition.

The phonetic inventories of 34 children between the ages of 15 and 24 months were investigated by Stoel-Gammon (1985). Although Stoel-Gammon's data demonstrated much individual variability, the results were compatible with some of the large-scale studies: they substantiated the early development of stops, nasals, and glides. In regard to the age of mastery for specific phonemes, Stoel-Gammon's findings were similar to Sander's (1972) data for phoneme mastery.

A longitudinal study of consonant production of seven children between the ages of 8 and 25 months by Robb and Bleile (1994) yielded results similar to Stoel-Gammon (1985). Both studies found children's initial-position consonants composed of voiced stops /b, d, g/ and nasals /m, n, ŋ/, then voiceless stops /p, t, k/ and fricatives /f, v, s, z/.

Most studies of typical speech development focus on singleton consonants rather than consonant clusters (e.g., /sp/, /tr/, /bl/). Some studies mention consonant cluster acquisition briefly (e.g., Arlt & Goodban, 1976; Bankson & Bernthal, 1990; Dyson, 1988; Haelsig & Madison, 1986; Poole, 1934; Stoel-Gammon, 1985; Wellman et al., 1931). Three key points that may be useful in assessment, analysis, or selection of appropriate intervention targets were identified by McLeod, van Doorn, and Reed (2001). First, word-final consonant clusters generally appear in inventories earlier than word-initial clusters (possibly related to the emergence of grammatical **morphemes**). Second, the acquisition of consonant clusters is gradual. Third, very young children typically delete one element of a consonant cluster (e.g., produce [tɑp] for *stop)* at first. Later, they may substitute for the previously missing element, until finally, the word is produced correctly.

How Can Norms Be Applied Clinically?

Most speech-language pathlogists (SLPs) rely on phoneme acquisition norms to make clinical decisions. Acquisition ages for specific phonemes vary from study to study, however. These inconsistencies are problematic when the data are used to determine eligibility for speech and language intervention services in the schools. Consequently, Porter and Hodson (2001) and a group of school-based speech-language pathologists conducted research to obtain phonological acquisition data for their own school district to assist in their remediation decisions. This investigation revealed general guidelines for them to use when creating goals and lessons for children on their caseloads. The 3-year-olds they studied had acquired all major phoneme classes except liquids /l, r/. Children between ages 4 and 5 acquired the /l/ phoneme, and those between 5 and 6 years acquired the /r/ phoneme. The results of this study can impact clinical decisions such as choosing sounds to focus on in intervention or deciding whether a child should receive intervention now or perhaps later.

Large-scale and longitudinal studies have been conducted to establish age norms for consonant development. Despite methodological difficulties and variability in individual phoneme acquisition, results of the studies concur that nasals, stops, and glides are acquired early; fricatives, affricates, and liquids are acquired later.

Patterns of Development

What Are Patterns of Speech Sound Development?

The information in the previous section addressed sound development for individual phonemes and sound classes. Some phonologists, however, are concerned with broad patterns of phonological acquisition (e.g., final consonants).

Several investigators have attempted to provide developmental data for the broad phonological patterns that characterize children's typical speech development. The term **phonological processes** (Ingram, 1976) has been used for error regularities (such as final consonant deletion) observed in children's speech productions; children learn to suppress processes that are inappropriate for their language. Although some similarities exist among the research, there are differences in the age that a phonological process is eliminated **(age of suppression)** and which processes occur more frequently at various ages. This section will provide an overview of research in phonological pattern acquisition and phonological process suppression.

Table 3.3

Grunwell's (1987) Chronology of Phonological Processes

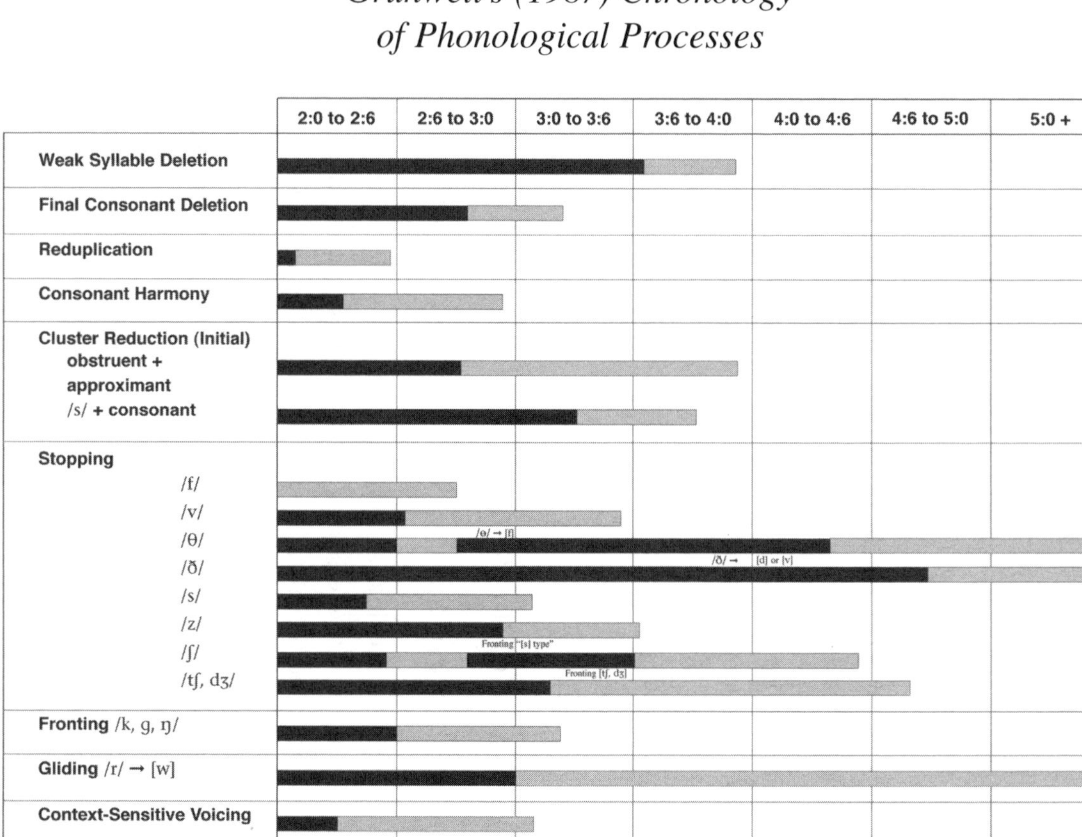

From *Clinical Phonology* (p. 183), by P. Grunwell, 1987, Gaithersburg, MD: Aspen Publishers. © 1987 by Aspen Publishers.

What Phonological Patterns/ Processes Occur in Typical Development?

Grunwell (1981, 1987) provides a chronology of phonological processes that identifies the duration and age of suppression for nine processes. Table 3.3 lists Grunwell's chronology. Final consonant deletion, for example occurs up to approximately 2:9 (2 years 9 months); then it begins to disappear and is likely eliminated by age 3:3. For clusters involving /s/ + consonant (e.g., /st/, /sp/), Grunwell found cluster reduction to be suppressed by age 3:3 and nonexistent by age 3:8.

The age of suppression of five phonological processes by 40 2-year-old children was examined by Dyson and Paden (1983). During the initial testing, the order for the frequency of process occurrence (from most to least) was found to be as follows: gliding, cluster reduction, fronting, stopping, and final-consonant deletion. During the final testing, at age 2:7, the order remained the same; however, final-consonant deletion was almost completely eliminated and fronting and stopping were infrequent. Gliding and cluster reduction were still common at age 2:7.

Preisser, Hodson, and Paden (1988) evaluated eight phonological processes in 60 children with typical development (ages 18–29 months). The most prevalent phonological processes evidenced by all children were cluster reduction and deviations involving liquids.

Haelsig and Madison (1986) investigated the occurrence of 16 phonological processes in 3-, 4-, and 5-year-old children to determine developmental criteria. Their results revealed that the processes of cluster reduction, weak syllable deletion, glottal replacement, labial assimilation, and gliding of liquids were used by 3- and 3½-year-old children, concluding that these processes should be expected in children at or under the age of 3. Weak syllable deletion and cluster reduction were prevalent in the speech of 4½- and 5-year-old children. Velar assimilation, prevocalic voicing, gliding of fricatives, affrication, and denasalization were rarely used by any age group. Haelsig and Madison found the greatest reduction in use of phonological processes occurred between 3 and 4 years of age.

Stoel-Gammon and Dunn (1985) presented a broad overview of speech acquisition with a model of the general stages of phonological development. Their

Table 3.4 *Stages of Phonological Development*

Prelinguistic Stage (1 month–1 year)	*First Words* (1 year–18 months)	*Phonemic Development* (18 months–4 years)	*Stabilization of the Phonological System* (4 years–8 years)
• Speech-like and nonspeech-like vocalizations • Speech-like vocalizations become prominent at the end of this stage	• Onset of meaningful words • Growth of vocabulary to 50 words • Productions are simple syllabic structure—CV, CVC, CVCV • Sounds are limited to stops, nasals, and glides	• Consonant clusters appear • Multisyllabic productions occur • Substitution patterns are common ([w] for /r/)	• Phonetic inventory completed • Exposure to reading and writing helps refine sound system

Source: Stoel-Gammon & Dunn (1985)

overview is presented in Table 3.4. As shown, the first two stages cover a relatively short age span. The last two stages consume nearly four years each. This model compiles findings from some of the studies already mentioned.

In addition to Stoel-Gammon and Dunn's (1985) overview, Hodson (1997) compiled phonological acquisition data from several studies to provide "flags" to indicate when to be concerned. Hodson's seven steps of phonological acquisition (see Table 3.5) serve as a guide to determine if a child's phonology is developing typically. Practitioners can compare a child's performance to that of children with typical development to ascertain if there is, indeed, a phonological impairment.

Although the data presented in this section can provide useful information for making clinical decisions, individual differences can have an impact on a child's speech sound development. The next section highlights work that has been done to study individual differences in phonological acquisition.

Table 3.5 *7 Steps of Phonological Acquisition*

Step	Age	Stage
1	1 year	Canonical babbling and vocables
2	1½ years	Recognizable words; CV structures; stops, nasals, glides
3	2 years	Final consonants, communication with words, "syllableness"
4	3 years	/s/ clusters, anterior-posterior contrasts, expansion of phonemic repertoire
5	4 years	Omissions rare, most "simplifications" suppressed, "adult-like" speech
6	5–6 years	Liquids /l/ (5 yrs) and /r/ (6 yrs), phonemic inventory stabilized
7	7 years	Sibilants and "th" perfected, "adult standard" speech

Source: Hodson (1997)

Individual Differences

Universal patterns cannot account for a child's phonological development in its entirety. Because no two people are exactly alike, it stands to reason that individual differences play a role in all aspects of development, including the development of the human speech sound system. No two children acquire their phonological system in precisely the same manner. Children employ idiosyncratic (i.e., unique) strategies that make their phonological system differ from others.

Several phonologists have examined individual differences in phonological development. The extent of individual variability can be remarkable. Children may differ in the sounds they produce, in the organization of their phonological system, and in their approaches to learning phonology (Vihman, 1998b).

Stoel-Gammon and Cooper (1984) and Vihman, Ferguson, and Elbert (1986) examined individual differences from the late babbling period through the acquisition of meaningful speech. Stoel-Gammon and Cooper analyzed the early lexical and phonological development in three children and found they differed significantly in these areas. Their vocal productions were most similar in the late babbling stage to the first-word stage. From then on, productions became more and more divergent (e.g., one child used many **phones** in the final position, while the other two children used very few). Vihman et al. collected data from 10 children (aged 9 to 16 months) and found individual variation predominated in the three areas they investigated (1) phonetic tendencies, (2) consonant inventory, and (3) word selection. Furthermore, results revealed that phonological processes typical of development from age 1 to 3 or 4 years were found to originate in the phonetic tendencies of the prelinguistic period.

Vihman and Greenlee (1987) studied individual differences in phonological acquisition of 10 children observed at 1 year and again at 3 years of age. The children were found to differ in intelligibility and in specific segment substitutions and cluster reductions. Although the children were from similar backgrounds, they differed considerably in rate of vocabulary acquisition and relative phonological maturity, as well as in their general learning style.

The phenomenon of phonological selection and avoidance in early **lexical acquisition** was examined by Schwartz and Leonard (1982). In previous studies, investigators (Ingram, 1976; Kiparsky & Menn, 1977) observed that young children were selective in the adult words they attempted; children followed a variety of individual patterns, selecting words with certain phonological characteristics and appearing to avoid words with other characteristics. Findings from the 12 children in the Schwartz and Leonard study concurred that young children are selective in the words they attempt, contingent upon their capabilities within their phonetic repertoires.

Phonetic preferences and word selection in two young girls were described by Vihman (1998b). These children, although matched for sex, socioeconomic status, amount of vocalization, and relative rate of lexical development, differed widely in their phonetic preferences, word selection, and stability of word shapes. One child demonstrated a preference for fricatives; the other preferred an unusually large number of words with final nasals. Differences were observed in their phonological organization. One child gradually increased the number of consonants that she attempted (restricting herself to mostly stops and nasals), whereas the other child used a broad array of consonants from the very beginning. The girls also differed in their choice of word shapes. One child's word productions were highly repetitive (i.e., producing many tokens of a single word type) with little variation, whereas the other child produced a different shape for almost every token of a given word.

Results of these studies demonstrate the range of variability that exists among children. For most children, these unique and idiosyncratic patterns gradually accommodate to the native language of the child, and eventually evolve into the adult sound system. But for the highly unintelligible child, individual differences may have an influence on the course of intervention.

Summary

Phonological acquisition is a complex process that begins at birth and extends into the early school-age years. Many factors affect the course of development. Several theorists have attempted to capture the origins of speech sound development.

Speech perception and babbling have been investigated extensively to unlock the mysteries of prelinguistic development. The transition from babbling to meaningful speech is important, leading the way for further phonological development. Numerous studies have tried to identify speech sound acquisition from various perspectives: individual phonemes, sound classes, and sound patterns. Guidelines have been established for phonological acquisition; however, a cookbook approach is not advisable. Individual differences must be taken into account.

PART II

Evaluation & Intervention Options

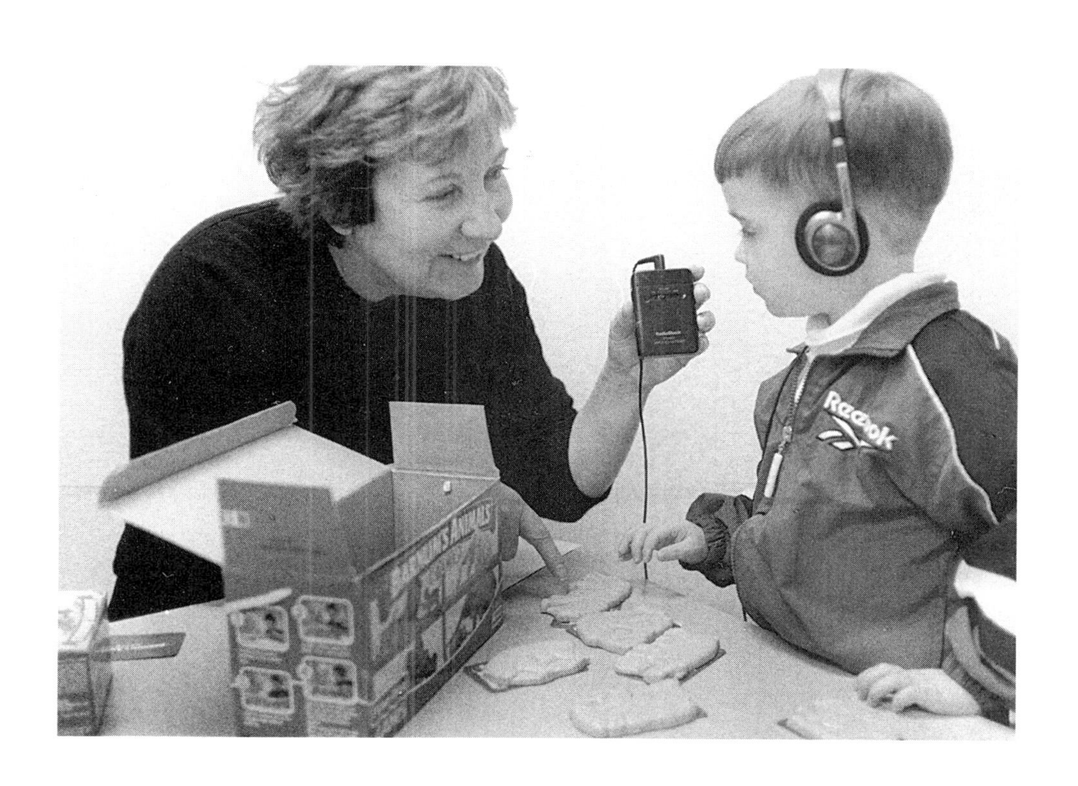

CHAPTER 4

Overview of the Diagnostic Evaluation Process for Children with Highly Unintelligible Speech

Barbara Williams Hodson

General Diagnostic Evaluation Considerations

- What Are the Major Goals of a Diagnostic Evaluation?
- What Method Is Fundamental?
- What Client Background Information Is Needed?
- What Major Areas Need to Be Assessed?

Phonological Evaluation

- What Types of Stimuli and Samples Are Used to Obtain Speech Production Data?
- What Basic Information Should a Phonological Evaluation Yield?
- What Are Major Options for Evaluating Phonological Systems?

Assessing & Analyzing Phonological Systems of Children with Highly Unintelligible Speech

- What Theories Have Influenced Our Phonological Assessment/Analysis Procedures?
- How Are Speech Samples of Children with Highly Unintelligible Speech Obtained?
- How Are Phonological Deviations Categorized?
- How Is Stimulability Assessed?

Summary

Diagnostic evaluation is the basis for everything that professionals do for clients in communication sciences and disorders (Bleile, 2002; Hodson, Scherz, & Strattman, 2002). Decisions regarding recommendations and intervention may not be optimal unless valid data are available from a thorough scientific investigation. Additionally, it is imperative to recognize that "diagnosis is ongoing." The diagnostic evaluation process must not be restricted to the short period of time when some formal tests are administered. Nonetheless, the initial evaluation can set the stage and provide basic data that can be used in the process of determining if the individual has a disorder and whether eligibility criteria (e.g., legal and school requirements) are met. In addition, results from the initial diagnostic evaluation often raise additional questions for consideration, and these may lead to referrals.

It is important to differentiate two basic evaluation-related processes: **screening** and in-depth diagnosis. **Screening** instruments and procedures provide only preliminary information that is used to determine if further in-depth testing (i.e., a diagnostic evaluation) is needed. Screening methods are used, as well, for initial testing of large numbers of children to find out which, if any, need further evaluation. In addition, some areas that are outside the scope of practice for speech-language pathologists (e.g., psychosocial behaviors) may be screened during diagnostic evaluation.

The first part of this chapter focuses on general aspects of a diagnostic evaluation for any child with a possible communication disorder. In the second part, options for phonological evaluations (e.g., type and size of speech sample) are discussed. The third section provides specific information about analyzing phonological systems of children with highly unintelligible speech. Although generic diagnostic evaluation information is included, the true focus of this chapter is on children with highly unintelligible speech.

General Diagnostic Evaluation Considerations

What Are the Major Goals of a Diagnostic Evaluation?

The primary goal of any diagnostic evaluation in communication sciences and disorders is to determine if there is, in fact, a **disorder/impairment.** The child's age, linguistic community, and existing conditions (e.g., fluctuating hearing acuity) must all be considered in this decision-making process. If assessment results indicate that a child's communication skills are below expectations, determining the level of **severity** (e.g., moderate, severe), which is a crucial component of any evaluation, is the second goal.

The third goal is to identify possible **etiological factors** that may predispose, precipitate, perpetuate, or even exacerbate existing conditions. A referral may need to be made for additional testing (e.g., to an audiologist) or for possible treatment (e.g., to an otolaryngologist). Two critical aspects need to be kept in mind when thinking about etiological factors. First, in many instances there are overlapping factors. Sometimes too much time is spent trying to differentially "eliminate" all but one etiological factor and then to assign a label, when in fact, several **concomitant** factors of varying degrees contribute to the difficulty. Second, it is important to think of a **continuum** of factors (e.g., different levels of hearing loss). Although an understanding of all etiological factors may not be critical for planning intervention, it is imperative to have a general knowledge base in order to determine prognosis.

A fourth goal of a diagnostic evaluation pertains to **prognosis.** For example, does the child have the potential for oral communication? If not, augmentative/alternative procedures need to be considered. If the prognosis is favorable (i.e., the child has the potential to communicate verbally), what are the expectations for communication?

The fifth goal, determining a direction for intervention, requires synthesis and integration of the outcomes of the four preceding goals. Information regarding evaluation results and recommendations for intervention, if indicated, as well as various options, need to be explained to caregivers.

What Method Is Fundamental?

The **scientific method** is an integral component of the diagnostic evaluation process. Based on observations, background information, and results of formal and informal testing, **hypotheses** are formulated. These hypotheses are then tested during the evaluation session and/or during the course of intervention. Hypotheses may be accepted, rejected, or modified. If the hypotheses are modified or if new hypotheses are formulated, these also need to be tested. For example, a common hypothesis for a child with highly unintelligible speech is that there is a major language impairment because children with highly unintelligible speech commonly omit morphological markers. If a child obtains a score that is within normal limits on a receptive language test (e.g., Test for Auditory Comprehension of Language [3rd ed.]; Carrow-Woolfolk, 1999), the hypothesis that the child has a pervasive language impairment would be rejected. The child's expressive language difficulties may be related to the child's phonological deviations (e.g., strident deficiencies may have an impact on morphological markers such as plurals). The process continues until hypotheses can be formulated and accepted based on scientific information.

What Client Background Information Is Needed?

First, clinicians need to know why the child has been referred for testing and by whom. It also is important to know if the child has had any prior speech-language evaluations or intervention services, and if so, what type, to what extent, and what the outcomes were. Information about the child's birth, as well as developmental and medical histories, should also be obtained. Although some of the information may not be pertinent, diagnosticians need to consider all possible etiological factors.

Among the physical factors that must be considered/evaluated are (1) syndromes, (2) sensory deficits (e.g., hearing loss), (3) structural anomalies (e.g., submucous cleft), and (4) neurophysiological involvement. Psychosocial factors, such as (1) environment, (2) culture, (3) emotional/motivational aspects, and (4) learning abilities and experiences, also need to be considered. In addition, knowing if any other languages are spoken in the child's home, to ascertain if deviations might be related to dialect, is important. Basic information about the child's cognitive abilities, as well as his or her general level of functioning, is also a relevant part of background information.

What Major Areas Need to Be Assessed?

If background information and/or results of phonological screening indicate that intelligibility is a primary concern, a comprehensive phonological evaluation is essential. A thorough description of phonological evaluation begins on page 51.

The second absolute requirement is hearing testing. A large percentage of children with intelligibility issues have histories of recurrent otitis media accompanied by fluctuating hearing loss. Minimal requirements for an audiological assessment for a child with highly unintelligible speech include pure-tone threshold testing and tympanometry.

The next area of primary concern for assessment is the child's language abilities. Information from caregivers, along with observation, can provide preliminary information about language skills and general functioning, but formal tests often need to be administered as well. If the child has highly unintelligible speech, expressive language assessment results are likely to be compromised. Moreover, language sample analyses usually cannot be completed until the child's level of intelligibility improves. Receptive language testing is necessary to determine if language problems exist beyond what would occur because of expressive phonological difficulties (e.g., comprehension). Another area that needs to be examined is pragmatics. Some children react to people not understanding them by withdrawing. Others react with frustration; consequently, there may be behavioral issues.

Structure and function of the oral mechanism also should be examined during a diagnostic evaluation. Typically, size and symmetry of the oral mechanism and movements of the lips, tongue, and velum are assessed. In addition, **diadochokinetic** rate (e.g., time required for 10 repetitions of /pʌtʌkʌ/) is often measured and compared to typical rates. Williams and Stackhouse (2000) found that accuracy and consistency of diadochokinetic responses were more sensitive than rate of responses when evaluating preschoolers. Notation should be made if noisy and/or mouth breathing is occurring. If screening results indicate that there are some areas of concern regarding the child's oral mechanism, a more in-depth evaluation of the structure and function (e.g., St. Louis & Ruscello, 2000) may be needed, as well as possible referrals (e.g., to an otorhinolaryngologist). As Bleile (2002) noted, however, "only gross abnormalities interfere with speech production" because the mechanism is "highly flexible and adaptable" (p. 248).

Because many children who are highly unintelligible experience difficulties in the areas of literacy, **phonological (or metaphonological) awareness** testing (e.g., rhyming, blending, segmenting) should be considered (see Chapter 8). This testing may be conducted either during the diagnostic evaluation session or later during remediation sessions.

If observations during conversation with the child indicate that there are voice, fluency, and/or prosody/suprasegmental issues, these aspects should be noted.

Further evaluation of each of these aspects of communication would then be indicated.

Stackhouse and Wells (1997) developed a comprehensive **psycholinguistic** assessment framework that is also useful for identifying levels of breakdown in speech processing. The psycholinguistic approach examines the child's speech problems as stemming from a "breakdown at one or more levels of input, stored linguistic knowledge, or output" (p. 7). The framework includes examining the child's input processing (skills necessary for decoding speech signals) and the child's output processing (skills necessary for encoding and producing speech). In this framework, the following six areas of input processing are examined.

1. Adequacy of hearing/auditory perception (e.g., hearing testing)
2. Ability to discriminate between real words (e.g., using words that are minimal pairs, such as *pea* and *bee)*
3. Ability to discriminate speech sounds without reference to lexical representations (i.e., which puppet said which nonword)
4. Existence of language-specific representations of word structures (e.g., determining illegal versus legal words)
5. Awareness of the internal structure of phonological representations (e.g., identifying pictures of words that rhyme)
6. Accuracy of phonological representations (e.g., blending of sound segments presented by examiner, such as /k/ /æ/ /t/, with the child then identifying the appropriate picture)

The following six areas, which pertain to the child's output processing (skills for encoding and producing speech), also are examined in the Stackhouse and Wells framework:

1. Adequacy of sound production skills (e.g., structure and function of oral mechanism)
2. Accuracy of motor programs (e.g., appropriate productions of sounds/sequences during pronunciations of words)
3. Accuracy of articulation of real words (e.g., spontaneous speech)

4. Accuracy of articulation of speech without reference to lexical representations (e.g., nonword repetition)

5. Manipulation of phonological units (e.g., **spoonerism**)

6. Rejection of one's own erroneous forms (e.g., self-correction)

According to Stackhouse and Wells, children with severe speech problems typically break down at more than one level, with both input and output often being involved.

Phonological Evaluation

What Types of Stimuli and Samples Are Used to Obtain Speech Production Data?

The first step for any phonological evaluation is to obtain a **speech sample** of some kind. Clinicians must first determine the type of speech sample needed.

Some phonologists (e.g., Shriberg & Kwiatkowski, 1980) require that a **continuous conversational speech sample** be obtained and analyzed. Stoel-Gammon and Dunn (1985), however, noted that (1) a continuous speech sample is usually more time consuming to collect and more difficult to transcribe than **single-word samples,** (2) unintelligible utterances cannot be analyzed, and (3) the range of phonemes attempted may be restricted. Additional problems arise when comparing scores over time because a child may produce quite dissimilar sets of words during different sampling times. In spite of these obstacles, it is recommended that a continuous speech sample be recorded during each evaluation so that samples can be compared over time. Pre- and post-intervention percentage measures of **intelligibility** can be derived from these samples.

Another procedure to obtain a speech sample is sentence imitation (e.g., Lowe, 1995). This method does yield a type of connected speech sample. Potential imitation effects, however, must be considered. Post-intervention scores might be inflated because children who have already received speech-language services tend to imitate words more accurately than when they say these words spontaneously. One other consideration is that some young children refuse to repeat sentences. Another method of obtaining a connected speech sample is oral reading for children who are already able to decode words.

The most common method for gathering a single-word sample is to use **stimuli** such as pictures (e.g., Bankson & Bernthal, 1990; Dodd, Hua, Crosbie, Holm, & Ozanne, 2003; Khan & Lewis, 2002; Secord & Donahue, 2002), or photographs (e.g., Smit & Hand, 1997). Our preference is to use objects (Hodson, 2004a) for elicitation. Most of our clients are preschoolers, who enjoy manipulating and naming objects. Perhaps even more important, we have found repeatedly that results obtained while children manipulate objects are more representative of a child's true level of performance. Children who have already received remediation tend to produce more sounds correctly while naming pictures—resulting in inflated post-intervention scores—than when they are manipulating and naming three-dimensional stimuli.

Another consideration pertains to size of the sample. Some phonologists (e.g., Grunwell, 1985) advocate analyzing an "exhaustive" speech sample of at least 200 words. The average time required for Grunwell's basic analysis procedure typically exceeds 15 hours. Such a procedure may be necessary for some research studies, but practitioners with large caseloads report they cannot spend that much time on any one procedure.

Our recommendation is that phonological assessment words include at least 10 opportunities for production of each of the major phonological deviations. In addition, the stimulus words should generally be familiar to preschool children. Additional prompts can be given, or when necessary, **delayed imitation** (i.e., naming the object, then saying a few other words before asking the child to give the name) may be employed for words that are not named readily. We advocate that more than one phonological deviation be assessed per word for efficiency purposes. Opportunities should be provided for productions of all consonants, most vowels and diphthongs, and common consonant clusters as well. In addition, it is important that some of the words be multisyllabic (see Larrivee & Catts, 1999).

What Basic Information Should a Phonological Evaluation Yield?

The essential requirement for clinical purposes is that an evaluation provide the following information:

1. A child's phonological **strengths** and **weaknesses**, including phonetic/phonemic and phonotactic (syllable shapes) **inventories**, as well as a measure of phonological deviations
2. The severity level of the disorder
3. A **direction for intervention,** including phonological **patterns** that need to be targeted
4. **Stimulability** results
5. Measures that can be used to **document changes** following intervention (i.e., **dynamic assessment** for **evidence-based practice**)

What Are Major Options for Evaluating Phonological Systems?

A **relational analysis** involves comparing a child's productions with that of adults in the linguistic community. An **independent analysis** focuses on the child's phonetic and phonotactic inventories independent of adult productions. It is not necessary to know what the child is attempting to say for an independent analysis, whereas relational analysis requires that the actual target word be known so that the "errors" can be compared with the target sounds.

Phoneme-Oriented Assessment Methods

Most norm-referenced speech sound assessment instruments (typically referred to as articulation tests) do not differentiate types of errors in the final tally. Specific sound errors are transcribed on a form, and substitutions, omissions, distortions, and additions (often referred to as SODA) are summarized in the resulting reports. Typically the score reported by both clinicians and researchers is based on the child's number of errors on the test. Distortions are counted as being equal to omissions, even though omissions have a more adverse effect on intelligibility than distortions.

Another phoneme-oriented measure that is commonly reported in the literature is the **Percentage of Consonants Correct (PCC;** Shriberg & Kwiatkowski, 1982). The formula for obtaining a child's PCC involves dividing the number of consonants produced correctly by the total number of consonants in the sample and then multiplying by 100. PCCs are assigned severity levels as follows:

> 85% (or normal) = Mild disorder
65–85% = Mild/Moderate disorder
50–65% = Moderate-to-Severe disorder
< 50% = Severe disorder

(NOTE: The PCC gives the same weighting to distortions as to substitutions and omissions.)

An extension of the PCC, the Percentage of Consonants Correct–Revised (PCC–R), scores omissions and substitutions as incorrect, but distortions are not counted as incorrect. There is no differentiation, however, in weighting between substitutions and omissions. Shriberg, Austin, Lewis, McSweeny, and Wilson (1997) stated that the PCC–R is the "most appropriate metric for comparisons involving speakers of diverse ages and of diverse speech status" (p. 720).

Methods Emphasizing Words

A method used for over 30 years is **Whole Word Accuracy (WWA**; McCabe & Bradley, 1975). WWA refers to the number of words in spontaneous conversation that are free from errors.

The method that is generally considered to be the most **valid** ecologically—is the **Percentage of Identifiable** (intelligible) **Words (PIW)** in a connected speech sample. To obtain a PIW, at least one unfamiliar listener writes the words that can be identified. The number of words identified is divided by the number of words in the sample and then multiplied by 100 to obtain the PIW (see Gordon-Brannan & Hodson, 2000, for additional information about this procedure).

A relatively new measure, **Phonological Mean Length of Utterance** (PMLU; Ingram & Ingram, 2001), does involve some differentiation between omissions and substitutions. One point is counted for each "segment" produced by the child (correct or incorrect—including vowels and syllabic consonants). One point is added for each correct consonant. Thus an omission results in the loss of 2 points, whereas a substitution is penalized 1 point. The sum of these two scores is then divided by the number of words in the sample. Longer words, therefore, result in extra points overall because more sounds are available for fewer words.

Linguistic Analysis Procedures

In the 1970s, speech-language practitioners began using **distinctive features** and **natural processes** to identify broader patterns of children's speech errors. (These analysis methods and also various **nonlinear** analyses are explained thoroughly by Edwards in Chapter 9. In addition, some influences of these linguistic analysis procedures are discussed in the next section of this chapter.)

Assessing & Analyzing Phonological Systems of Children with Highly Unintelligible Speech

What Theories Have Influenced Our Phonological Assessment/Analysis Procedures?

Distinctive feature analysis and phonological rule writing based on **generative phonology** (Chomsky & Halle, 1968) were the first steps into phonologically based clinical analyses. Phonological rules were useful, but they did not lead directly to the identification of broad target patterns for intervention goals. Although distinctive feature analysis provides information regarding feature differences between a child's substitution (e.g., – continuant) and the target sound in a word (e.g., + continuant), it has one critical limitation: Distinctive feature analysis does not account for omissions, an extremely common phenomenon in utterances of children with highly unintelligible speech.

Phonological process analysis (Ingram, 1976), based on **Natural Phonology Theory** (Stampe, 1972), became popular in the late 1970s and early 1980s (e.g., Shriberg & Kwiatkowski, 1980; Weiner, 1979). Broad patterns could be identified readily both for omissions (e.g., cluster reduction) and for common substitutions (e.g., fronting), as well as for many other phonological "processes" (e.g., assimilations). The initial goal of natural phonology intervention was to teach children to "suppress" innate simplification processes. One of the limitations of natural process analysis is that children with highly unintelligible speech often demonstrate unusual deviations (e.g., backing, initial consonant deletion) that are not "natural" simplifications. Moreover, typical phonological process analyses do not lead directly to specification of deficient phoneme classes that need to be targeted.

Specific categories of consonants (e.g., velars, stridents) need to be assessed directly, rather than just noting numbers of simplification processes (e.g., 10 occurrences of fronting) that affect them because of overlapping **constituent** processes. For example, a highly unintelligible child who has extensive omissions, including velars, might not evidence fronting at all because of its being "blocked" by omissions (e.g., final consonant deletion). In fact, scores for substitution processes such as fronting sometimes increase during a re-evaluation even when a child's overall phonological system and intelligibility clearly are improving. This phenomenon occurs because substitutions often replace omissions temporarily until the child learns to produce the actual target consonants. For example, it is not uncommon for a child to say /wɑ/ for *rock* during the first evaluation, /wɑt/ during another assessment, and /wɑk/ at a later time. Major consonant categories need to be assessed explicitly in order to determine exactly which categories of consonants, as well as syllable structures, need to be targeted.

The culmination of some 30 years of clinical research and practice involving several hundred children with highly unintelligible speech has resulted in the Hodson Assessment of Phonological Patterns–3rd edition (HAPP–3; Hodson, 2004a). The HAPP–3 is not totally aligned with any one theory. Rather, it incorporates components that are compatible with several phonological theories. For example, some distinctive feature classes (e.g., stridents) are assessed. Moreover, some remnants of natural phonology simplification substitution processes (e.g., stopping, gliding) still remain. In addition, some HAPP–3 categories (e.g., velar, singleton postvocalic consonant omission) are comparable to nonlinear phonology categories (e.g., dorsal, prosodic).

How Are Speech Samples of Children with Highly Unintelligible Speech Obtained?

The primary goal of phonological assessment is to help speech-language practitioners obtain data as expeditiously as possible, thus providing a framework for designing efficient and effective individualized intervention plans. We use objects (e.g., *spoon),* questions (e.g., How many *crayons* are there?), and a few pictures (e.g., *smoke)* to elicit 50 spontaneous naming responses and a continuous speech sample. The child's productions are transcribed at the time of utterance and then verified by playing and replaying audio recordings.

How Are Phonological Deviations Categorized?

Phonological Deviations (e.g., **Omissions, Major Substitutions)** that have been observed in children's utterances are listed in Table 4.1. Other deviations/distortions **(Minimal Place of Articulation Shifts)** are provided in Table 4.2 (page 63). Explanations of these deviations and some examples are provided in the following sections, with examples for all being provided in the tables.

Omissions of Sound Segments

Syllables

There are three major types of syllable omissions. The first involves reducing the number of syllables in a word to one syllable. Some children experience considerable

Table 4.1 *Major Phonological Deviations in Children's Utterances*

Omissions	
Syllables • Reductions to monosyllables • Weak syllable deletion (typical) • Multisyllabicity problems	 basket → [bæ____] remember → [__mɛmbɚ] extinguisher → [ɛ_stɪŋg____ɚ]
Singleton Consonants • Postvocalic (word-final) • Intervocalic (word-medial) • Prevocalic (word-initial)	 boat → [boʊ_] bucket → [bʌ_ət] boat → [_oʊt]
Consonant Sequences/Clusters • Reductions • Deletions	 truck → [t_ʌk] truck → [__ʌk]
Major Substitutions	
Fronting (posterior → anterior)	key → [ti]
Backing (anterior → posterior)	tea → [ki]
Stopping	leaf → [dip]
Gliding	leaf → [jif]
Vowelization	zipper → [zipʊ]
Palatalization	see → [ʃi]
Depalatalization	she → [si]
Affrication	shoe → [tʃu]
Deaffrication	chew → [ʃu]

Continued on next page

Table 4.1—Continued

Major Assimilations	
Labial (regressive and progressive)	spoon → [fpum]
Velar	duck → [gʌk]
Alveolar	duck → [dʌt]
Palatal	juice → [ʤuʃ]
Nasal	bone → [mon]
Liquid	yellow → [lɛlo]
Glottal Stop Replacement	
Omitted Segment	boat → [boʊʔ]
Dialectal	button → [bʌʔn̩]
Syllable-Structure/Context-Related Changes	
Metathesis	mask → [mæks]
Migration	smoke → [moʊks]
Coalescence	smoke → [foʊk]
Reduplication	basket → [bæbæ]
Epenthesis	blue → [bəlu]
Diminutive	sheep → [ʃipi]
Cluster Creation	soap → [stoʊp]
Voicing Alterations	
Prevocalic Voicing	cup → [gʌp]
Prevocalic Devoicing	gum → [kʌm]
Postvocalic Devoicing (normal)	page → [peɪʧ]
Postvocalic Voicing (rare)	leaf → [liv]
Vowel Alterations	
Neutralization	bed → [bɑd]
Dialectal	eye → [ɑ]
Idiosyncratic Rules	
Child Preferences	kitty → [ʃɪʃi]

Adapted from *Targeting Intelligible Speech* (2nd ed.; p. 37), by B. Hodson & E. Paden, 1991, Austin, TX: Pro-Ed. © 1991 by Barbara Williams Hodson and Elaine Pagel Paden. Adapted with permission.

difficulty producing more than one syllable at a time or they might repeat the same syllable. The child who reduces all words to **monosyllables** is extremely difficult to understand. The second type of syllable omission—**weak syllable** deletion—is common in adults as well as children and is not considered to be a disorder. The third type of syllable omission pertains to **multisyllabic** words. Most children are able to produce multisyllabic words appropriately by the age of 6 years (Jenkins,

1988). Some individuals, however, have difficulty producing all of the syllables and all of the sounds in complex multisyllabic words.

Singleton Consonants

Singleton consonant omission can be postvocalic, prevocalic, or intervocalic. **Postvocalic** singleton consonant omission (also referred to as final consonant deletion, open syllable, or CV preference) is common in the speech of toddlers (around the age of 18 months) and in the utterances of children with disordered expressive phonological systems. **Prevocalic** singleton consonant omission is much less common unless a child uses only vowels. Children typically produce consonant-vowel (CV) structures by the age of 12 months, although substitutions are common because of their limited phonetic repertoire. **Intervocalic** singleton consonant omissions occur when children delete word-medial singleton consonants. Some children produce word beginnings and word endings, but no consonants in between.

Consonant Sequences/Clusters

The term **consonant sequence** refers to all contiguous consonants (e.g., /θbr/ in *toothbrush),* whereas **consonant cluster** refers to adjacent consonants in the same syllable (i.e., /br/). Consonant sequence/cluster **reduction,** which is an extremely common phonological deviation among children with highly unintelligible speech (see Hodson & Paden, 1981), occurs when one consonant (or more) in a sequence is omitted with at least one consonant remaining; deletion refers to omission of all of the consonants in the sequence.

Major Substitutions

Fronting

Fronting refers to the substitution of an anterior consonant for a posterior one. Fronting is fairly common in utterances of children with expressive phonological impairments. Anterior consonants include /p, b, m, w, t, d, s, z, n, l, f, v, θ, ð/; posterior consonants include /k, g, ŋ, h/.

Backing

Backing involves the reverse direction of substitution. A posterior consonant is substituted for an anterior one. Backing, which is much less common than fronting, seems to have a particularly adverse effect on intelligibility.

Stopping

Stopping refers to the substitution of a stop (/p, b, t, d, k, g/) for a "nonstop" (i.e., fricatives, nasals, glides, liquids) consonant. Stopping is fairly common in utterances of children with an expressive phonological impairment (EPI).

Gliding

Gliding occurs when children substitute /w/ or /j/ for another consonant, most commonly for liquids. Gliding is fairly common in utterances of preschool children.

Vowelization

Vowelization refers to the production of a pure vowel in the place of a vocalic liquid. The term "vocalization" is used by many phonologists for this phenomenon, but clinicians report some confusion with the term **infant vocalizations.** Liquid vowelization also is fairly common in the speech of young children with typical phonological development.

Palatalization/Depalatalization

Palatalization and depalatalization refer to the addition or loss of the palatal component, particularly for sibilants. When a child says [ʃi] for *see,* palatalization has occurred; [si] for *she* is depalatalization.

Affrication/Deaffrication

Affrication and deaffrication refer to the addition or loss of the combination of stop and fricative. Thus [tʃu] for *shoe* is affrication. [ʃu] or [tu] for *chew* is deaffrication, with the latter example, [tu], also involving depalatalization.

Major Assimilations

Assimilation involves altering a phoneme so that it takes on a characteristic of another sound in the word, even if that sound has been omitted. Some assimilations are common in adult speech as well as in the speech of children with EPI. For example, we say [bæŋk] for *bank.* Substitutions that on first inspection may appear to be inconsistent are often byproducts of assimilation. For example, if a child says [to] for *so,* but [po] for *soap,* most likely the /p/ for /s/ is an artifact of assimilation even though word-final /p/ was omitted. Regressive **assimilation** affects a sound earlier in the word; progressive **assimilation** influences a later sound.

Labial assimilation is fairly common in the speech of young children. For example, many preschoolers with typical development say [fwɪm] for *swim.* Children with EPI, however, often use labial assimilation excessively (e.g., [po] for *soap;* [pwin] for *queen).* Velar assimilation occurs when a velar is produced for a nonvelar sound because of another velar in the target word. **Velar** assimilation also occurs in the speech of some preschoolers with typical development (e.g., [gɔgi] for *doggie).* **Alveolar** assimilation occurs when a child substitutes an alveolar consonant because of another alveolar in the word. Alveolar assimilation can be differentiated from fronting by having the child say two words, one with an alveolar (e.g., *cat)* and one without (e.g., *car).* If the child substitutes /t/ in both instances, it can be assumed that fronting is an overriding deviation. But if the child substitutes /t/ only for /k/ in *cat,* this would be alveolar assimilation. There are many types of assimilation. Three other fairly common types are **palatal, nasal,** and **liquid** (see Table 4.1 on pages 57–58 for examples).

Glottal Stop Replacement

Some children "mark" final consonants by substituting a glottal stop until they are able to produce word endings. Children with palatal anomalies (e.g., repaired cleft palate) often produce glottal stops excessively. Glottal stops sometimes are produced because of dialects (e.g., Scottish English) and also specific contexts (e.g., *button* → [bʌʔn̩]).

Syllable-Structure/Context-Related Changes

Metathesis and **migration** involve changes in word positions. Metathesis occurs when two phonemes or syllables exchange places. For migration, only one sound moves. **Coalescence** is observed when two phonemes are replaced by one phoneme that has characteristics of the original two sounds, but is neither of the original sounds. **Reduplication** refers to the repetition of phonemes or syllables. This occurs commonly in the speech of toddlers as they are learning to sequence two or more syllables. **Epenthesis** occurs when there is a sound addition. A common example is the insertion of the schwa (/ə/) between two consonants in a cluster. **Diminutive** is an endearing pattern that varies with the language. In English, we often add /i/ to nouns when speaking to toddlers (e.g., *horsie).* **Cluster creation** occurs when a second consonant is added to a singleton (e.g., [sti] for *see).*

Voicing Alterations

Prevocalic voicing is fairly common in utterances of children with highly unintelligible speech. **Postvocalic devoicing** is extremely common in the speech of children with typical phonological development and also adults. **Prevocalic devoicing** is much less common than the first two types of voicing alterations, and **postvocalic voicing** is extremely rare.

Vowel Alterations

Many vowel differences are related to **dialects** (e.g., Southern American). Some children with highly unintelligible speech produce only a few vowels (e.g., /ɑ/), with other vowels and diphthongs being **neutralized** to these.

Idiosyncratic Rules/Child Preferences

Sometimes children have individual preferences that cannot be categorized as any of the above deviations. Some have a preferred sound that they substitute for most sounds. Others may restrict these substitutions to certain positions in words.

Other Deviations/Distortions

The deviations listed in Table 4.2 can be disturbing to a listener, but typically these deviations alone do not have a particularly adverse effect on intelligibility. **Minimal place of articulation shifts,** such as substitutions of some anterior stridents (e.g., /f/) for the interdental fricatives, often cannot be identified unless the listener sees the child's mouth. The same is true for the **frontal/interdental lisp** in the speech of preschoolers. Stridency is maintained, but the tongue placement is forward. The **lateral lisp** can, of course, be heard, but it is not a phonemic difference (i.e., does not result in a change in meaning). **Tongue protrusions** for other alveolar consonants also must be seen to be identified. **Nasalization** is another nonphonemic alteration that sometimes is related to oral structure difficulties (e.g., velopharyngeal incompetence). There are many other types of distortions that are found in the speech of children with repaired cleft palates (e.g., pharyngealization).

Table 4.2 *Other Deviations/Distortions*

Minimal Place ofArticulation Shifts (Phonemic)	
/f, v, s, z/ for "th"	*teeth* → [tif]
Minimal Place ofArticulation Shifts (Phonetic)	
Lisps for sibilants (stridency maintained) • Frontal/interdental • Lateral lisp	 *see* → [s̟i] *see* → [s͍i]
Other tongue protrusions	*note* → [n̟oʊt̟]
Nasalization	*see* → [sĩ]

Adapted from *Targeting Intelligible Speech* (2nd ed.; p. 37), by B. Hodson & E. Paden, 1991, Austin, TX: Pro-Ed. © 1991 by Barbara Williams Hodson and Elaine Pagel Paden. Adapted with permission.

How Is Stimulability Assessed?

After the child's phonological system has been analyzed, phonemes, including consonant clusters, that were not produced in any word position should be identified. These phonemes/clusters then need to be evaluated for **stimulability,** which refers to the ability to produce the sound correctly when modeling and assistance are provided. The examiner typically starts with modeling. If the child cannot imitate the sound, additional assists are added (e.g., tactile cues, amplification). See Appendix B for suggestions on eliciting consonant productions. Notations need to be made regarding the techniques that led to appropriate productions, as well as to specify those phonemes that were not stimulable during the examination.

Summary

The general goal for this chapter has been to review phonological assessment/ analysis options in the context of evaluating children who are highly unintelligible. This has been done in order to assist clinicians in the process of making informed decisions when planning and conducting diagnostic examinations. General information about the overall diagnostic evaluation process in communication sciences and disorders also was discussed. In addition, specific information about assessing and analyzing the speech of children with highly unintelligible speech was provided, and phonological deviations that have been observed in children's utterances were described.

CHAPTER 5

Overview of Intervention Approaches, Methods & Targets

Kathy Strattman

Intervention Approaches

Early Intervention Approaches

- What Was the Focus in Early Phoneme-Oriented Intervention?
- What Is the Emphasis for Phonetic Placement?
- What Did the Moto-Kinesthetic Approach Add?
- What Are the Steps in the Stimulus Approach?
- How Is Coarticulation Utilized in the Sensory-Motor Approach?
- What Is the Focus of the Discrimination Approach?

Behavioristic Programs

- How Is a Behavioristic Program Implemented?
- How Is Programmed Instruction Used?
- How Are Instructional Objectives Written?
- What Are Intervention Targets for the Multiple Phonemic Approach?

Linguistic-Based Approaches

- How Are Distinctive Features Incorporated in Intervention?
- What Is the Goal of Phonologically Based Approaches?
- What Is Targeted in the Cycles Approach?
- How Is the Metaphon Approach Used to Develop Reorganization of the Sound System?
- How Does Phonological Awareness Influence Expressive Phonology?
- How Can a Whole Language Approach Affect Expressive Phonology?

Target Selection Considerations

Targets for Phoneme-Oriented Approaches

- How Are Target Phonemes Selected?

Targets for Contrast Approaches

- What Is the Target Focus of Minimal Pairs?
- What Is the Target Focus of Maximal Oppositions?
- What Is the Target Focus of Multiple Oppositions?

Targets for Patterned-Oriented Approaches

- How Are Targets Patterns Selected?

Summary

In conversation, the listener rarely notices pronunciation of individual sounds. It is only when sounds deviate from the expected sounds that attention is drawn to them—most especially if those deviations interfere with communication (Van Riper, 1939). The purpose of this chapter is to trace the evolution of speech sound intervention through descriptions of representative approaches. Many of these approaches are still used today. Wherever possible, additional references that describe the specifics of how to implement these approaches are provided. The chapter is divided into two sections: (1) Intervention Approaches and (2) Target Selection Considerations. In the first section, major approaches for intervention of speech sound deviations are summarized, including salient points of each approach, their implementations, and current practices. The emphasis in early intervention approaches was on correction of articulation deficiencies. Later, phoneme-oriented approaches reflected the influence of behaviorism. More recently, professionals have used linguistic-based approaches both to understand children's phonological development and to facilitate reorganization of their phonological systems. In the second section, the focus is on selection of remediation targets.

Intervention Approaches

Early Intervention Approaches

What Was the Focus in Early Phoneme-Oriented Intervention?

The title of a 1939 textbook by Charles Van Riper—*Speech Correction: Principles and Methods*—exemplified the clinical focus of the profession as it began. At that time, speech-language pathologists (SLPs) were called speech correctionists. Emphasis was on the "correction" of any communication deficiency, especially correction of the articulation of speech sounds that were different from conventional productions. The term **articulation** refers to the motor or movement components of sounds in terms of visual, auditory, and kinesthetic changes. The physical production of individual phonemes was emphasized in the major early intervention approaches, which included the following:

- Phonetic Placement
- Moto-Kinesthetic
- Stimulus
- Sensory-Motor
- Discrimination

In these approaches, one phoneme was treated at a time, and the intervention focused on the phonetic properties that were necessary for production and acoustic perception.

What Is the Emphasis for Phonetic Placement?

The Phonetic Placement Approach (Scripture & Jackson, 1927) is generally considered a traditional approach. In this approach, two things are emphasized: the placement of the articulators (e.g., tongue, lips) and the modification of the airstream for production of individual phonemes. The premise is that an individual does not articulate sounds correctly, because of inappropriate placement of the articulators and/or inappropriate modification of the airstream.

Intervention includes teaching appropriate placement of the articulators by physically assisting placement (e.g., touching the alveolar ridge with a tongue depressor) and appropriate modification of the airstream, also by assisting physical production (e.g., the use of straws to direct the breath stream). The production of the sound is demonstrated and described (e.g., for /t/, "Touch the alveolar ridge with your tongue tip, build up air pressure, and let air pop out over your tongue tip"). In addition, diagrams and demonstrations—including hand analogies (Paget, 1963), where one hand represented the teeth and palate and the other represent the tongue—could show position of the articulators and their movement. Considerable repetitive practice is required; generalization of static placement to dynamic speaking was challenging.

Today, the phonetic placement approach may still be useful in early phases of articulation intervention to demonstrate how a phoneme is produced. (See Bleile, 2004, for specific phonetic placement techniques.) The assumption in this approach is that phonemes are always articulated with the same placement and production. Phoneme productions do vary, however. Consider the tongue placement for /l/ in *lake* (alveolar tongue tip placement), from the /l/ in *bell* (farther back, often with pitch change). Productions shift slightly because of **coarticulation** to accommodate production of surrounding phonemes.

What Did the Moto-Kinesthetic Approach Add?

Speech is not a series of static positions, but a dynamic event. Sound production relies on a motoric process of shaping or obstructing exhaled air as it passes through the oral or nasal cavities. The Moto-Kinesthetic approach (Stinchfield & Young, 1938) involved external manipulation of the articulators. The premise is that this articulatory movement must be "felt" and developed as a muscle sense or kinesthetic image for monitoring correct placement in sound production.

The clinician's manipulations indicate where sounds occur or where articulators touch, thus facilitating the feeling of the articulatory movement (Bosley, 1981). An association is made between that feeling and the simultaneous auditory model provided by the clinician. In the Moto-Kinesthetic approach (Stinchfield & Young, 1938), the client lies on his or her back during the procedure to facilitate muscle relaxation. Initially, sounds are produced in syllables, beginning with the target sound and the schwa vowel. Production of reduplicated syllables, multisyllabic words, phrases, and then sentences follow.

Tactile cuing is part of the Moto-Kinesthetic approach. Tactile or touching cues continue to be useful in remediation to establish target sounds (e.g., tapping the upper lip to suggest tongue movement to the alveolar ridge to elicit /t/, or pressing up under the chin to stimulate raising the back of the tongue to touch the soft palate when eliciting /k/).

What Are the Steps in the Stimulus Approach?

Van Riper's Stimulus Approach (1939, 1947, 1954, 1963, 1972, 1978; Van Riper & Emerick, 1984; Van Riper & Erickson, 1996) is also referred to as a "traditional approach." Van Riper, however, viewed misarticulations as more than placement or production errors. He viewed poor auditory sensory perception as a contributing factor in misarticulations. He advocated auditory or ear training prior to production practice of individual sounds to stimulate the sensory perception of the phoneme. Van Riper acknowledged that individual phonemes vary within a phonetic context; however, he stressed that to later be integrated into conversational speech, a sound must first be said clearly in isolation. To avoid confusing a child, only one sound (and possibly the sound's voiced/voiceless **cognate** (e.g., /k/ and /g/) is targeted at a time.

The Stimulus Approach includes five steps with phases in each. The five steps are outlined below. For a more detailed information on the Stimulus Approach, see Van Riper and Emerick (1984).

1. **Sensory-Perceptual Training** (Ear Training) includes four phases:
    - Naming of the target sound using a descriptive cue (e.g., /s/ "snake" sound or /f/ "mad kitty" sound)
    - Identification of the position of the sound in a word, phrase, or sentence (e.g., beginning, middle, or end of a word)
    - Auditory stimulation using the target sound in a variety of activities (e.g., tongue twisters and sound-loaded sentences; *She sells sea shells by the seashore* for /s/)
    - Discrimination of the "new" target sound from the client's errors

2. Sound **elicitation** is established through any or all of the following:
   - Imitation (repeating the clinician's model)
   - Phonetic placement
   - Use of a mirror
   - Drawings of side views of the face
   - Static placement of tongue, teeth, lips, and velum
   - Moto-kinesthetic training
   - Sound approximation
3. Sound production is stabilized following an articulation hierarchy:
   - Isolated sound production (e.g., /s/)
   - Production in syllables with the target in the initial (/si/), final (/is/), and medial (/isi/) position of a word
   - Production of the target in all positions in single words (e.g., *see, bus, messy)*
   - Production of the target in short phrases (e.g., *see him)*
   - Production of the target sound in sentences *(The bus is late)*
4. **Transfer** of the sound production to other settings and **carryover** of the sound in conversational speaking are facilitated through speech assignments at home, school, or in the community; self-monitoring; and practice with various conversational partners in various settings.
5. **Maintenance** of the new correct production is promoted through follow-up sessions beginning weekly, later monthly, and finally every 6 months until dismissal.

Some SLPs use the Stimulus Approach today, especially for children with one or two speech sound errors. Descriptive cues and steps for transfer/carryover, and maintenance are often used. There is concern, however, that focusing on one target phoneme at a time is inefficient when many sounds are deficient. Also, considerable time may be spent just listening before actual production practice begins. In this approach, there is limited emphasis on generalization to untargeted phonemes.

How Is Coarticulation Used in the Sensory-Motor Approach?

In early phoneme-oriented approaches, the production of individual phonemes included attention to the position of the target sounds in words (i.e., initial, medial, or final positions). Production of sounds varies, however, as they are coarticulated with other phonemes (McDonald, 1964). McDonald viewed speech as a sequence of syllables, rather than as sounds in individual words. Phonemes could release syllables (e.g., /ti/) or arrest syllables (e.g., /it/). McDonald recommended using assessment procedures to examine coarticulation, that is, to "deep" test for coarticulation. For example, for /s/, he assessed consonant production before /s/ (e.g., *book sun)* and after /s/ (e.g., *bus book).*

McDonald's (1964) premise was that one context of coarticulation could facilitate consonant production in other positions. The goal was to discover the best contexts.

The Sensory-Motor Approach followed this sequence, using syllable productions:

- Heightened awareness of the "ballistic" speech movement patterns through bisyllable and trisyllable productions
- Correct production of sound sequences
- Correct production in varied phonetic contexts

Coarticulatory contexts using a key word (e.g., *book* for /k/) were used before or after the target phoneme (e.g., /s/ as described above) to facilitate correct productions. This approach did not include ear training or productions of phonemes in isolation.

Today, the Sensory-Motor Approach is considered to be useful in determining facilitative phonetic environments for coarticulation, especially for a phoneme that is difficult to elicit (e.g., /r/). Clinicians may occasionally do "deep" testing to investigate coarticulation effects that will facilitate correct production. Shine and Proust (1982) adapted McDonald's (1964) Sensory-Motor Approach, adding more structured phases in a behavioristic program.

What Is the Focus of the Discrimination Approach?

As mentioned previously, Van Riper (1934) advocated sensory-perceptual training through ear training. Based on that early premise, Winitz and Bellerose (1962) focused on teaching a child to discriminate the error sound from the target sound prior to target production. They believed that the ability to hear the difference between the correct sound and the error sound was the first step to correcting speech sound errors.

Winitz (1975) later suggested beginning discrimination tasks with word contrasts that were quite dissimilar (e.g., if /ʃ/ was produced as /ʧ/, the contrasts *ship/lock* were used), rather than contrasting the error sound with the correct sound (e.g., *ship/chip).* Winitz proposed that the initial use of gross contrasts would teach children to discriminate more easily, and then finer contrasts could be introduced later.

There has been controversy about whether or not discrimination tasks are necessary (Monnin, 1984). Discrimination tasks require **metalinguistic skills**—the ability to think and talk about word structures as opposed to word meaning. Younger children might not be able to discriminate their error sounds from correct production.

Behavioristic Programs

How Is a Behavioristic Program Implemented?

In a behavioristic program, the SLP determines target phonemes based on standardized speech sound testing. Baseline measures for all error phonemes are determined following an **"articulation hierarchy"** (e.g., production at the word level, elicited by 10–20 picture cards with the phoneme in at least the initiating [initial] and arresting [final] position in stimulus words). If a child can produce the sound correctly at the word level, **baseline** measures are checked at the phrase level and on up through the hierarchy. If a child cannot produce the sound correctly in words, baseline measures are obtained in isolation and then in nonsense syllables (CV, VC, and CVC). Behavioral objectives are written for each phoneme target, beginning with the level above the baseline measure. For example, if a child can produce /k/ with 90% accuracy in the initial, medial, and final positions of words elicited by picture cards, the next objective would be correct production of /k/ in phrases. Intervention follows this hierarchy. Movement up the levels requires the child to meet specified criterion levels, usually written in percentages. Reinforcement schedules are used for correct productions, and modifications or branches for breaking the task down (e.g., more prompting or selected words) are followed if productions are consistently incorrect. Transfer or generalization to nontreated words that initially contained errors is tested to determine progress.

How Is Programmed Instruction Used?

In the 1970s, educators and SLPs, responding to needs for efficiency and to document the effectiveness of intervention, were influenced by behaviorism (also referred to as behavior modification). Two popular behavioristic phoneme-oriented programs that emerged during the 1970s were Programmed Instruction (Mowrer, 1977) and the Multiple Phonemic Approach (McCabe & Bradley, 1975). These programs followed an articulation hierarchy, but responses were modified using specific reinforcement for correct sound productions and "penalties" for incorrect productions. Clinicians spent considerable time charting and tracking productions to reach a predetermined level of correct productions or **criterion.**

Mowrer, Baker, and Schutz (1968) followed behavior modification principles to develop the Programmed Instruction Approach for articulation. As mentioned earlier, in behavior modification, correct responses are elicited and shaped by consequences: reinforcement and penalty. SLPs followed programs that specified stimuli and antecedent events (e.g., modeling, prompting, and cuing).

Reinforcement schedules, including tangible (e.g., stickers) and token (e.g., poker chips) reinforcement for each correct sound production are a required part of intervention to establish consistent correct productions. Intermittent reinforcement (e.g., reinforcing every 10th correct response) follows after the client has met the criterion. Systematic penalties are specified to discourage or extinguish incorrect responses.

How Are Instructional Objectives Written?

Objectives that specify observable behavior are required. Objectives need to include (1) what the child is to do (e.g., *produce /k/ correctly in the word-final position*), (2) how or under what conditions (e.g., *when elicited by picture cards)*, and (3) at what criterion (e.g., *with 90% accuracy for two consecutive sessions)*. Although session planning follows a prescribed pattern, considerable time is spent in daily tracking and charting to demonstrate how objectives are being met.

Certainly, the efficiency of behavioristic programs and the data demonstrating progress are attractive; however, the concept of controlling human behavior with stimulus/reinforcement programming remains controversial. Programs are inflexible and not child centered. Many, many responses are required, making sessions tedious. The same intervention protocol for every session can be uninteresting for clients. Nonetheless, behavioristic methods are still incorporated by many SLPs today, especially those whose education was heavily influenced by behaviorism. Intervention objectives, which have become requirements for **individualized education programs (IEPs),** attention to antecedent stimuli, and reinforcement remain important components in most intervention approaches. In 1989, Mowrer wrote, "We needed the boost we received from the behaviorists during the 1960s and 1970s but, having learned these techniques, we perhaps are challenged to go on to other aspects of articulation" (p. 189).

What Are Intervention Targets for the Multiple Phonemic Approach?

The Multiple Phonemic Approach (McCabe & Bradley, 1975) is a programmed approach that is similar in structure to Programmed Instruction, but there are marked differences in selection of remediation targets. A general concern about the traditional approaches was efficiency. Children who were unintelligible could be in remediation for years when phonemes were treated singly, until each was carried over into conversational speaking. Some techniques used in the Multiple Phonemic Approach are similar to the Stimulus Approach, but the intervention targets are the opposite of the traditional single-phoneme target: All phonemes are targets.

The Multiple Phonemic Approach involves three phases: Establishment, Transfer, and Maintenance. There are multiple steps in each phase (e.g., six steps in Phase Two). Children can be at a different phase or step for different phonemes. Careful charting is required to track which phonemes are at which phase/step of intervention. The type of stimulus, response criterion, and reinforcement schedule are also programmed for each step, with specified branching steps that modify stimuli and reinforcement used when a criterion is not met. McCabe and Bradley (1975) stressed that intervention should focus on success, beginning and ending with production of sounds produced correctly.

In Phase One, **Establishment,** the goal is correct production of each consonant phoneme in isolation. Even phonemes the child already articulates correctly are elicited by graphemes written on cards to ensure success from the beginning. If time or the number of errors does not allow intervention, phonemes remain in a "holding" procedure in Phase One by practicing each sound correctly one time during each intervention session.

Phase Two, **Transfer,** also is similar to the Stimulus Approach. Phonemes are targeted in an articulation hierarchy. Branching is used for more specific practice if the criterion is not met. In Step 4, **whole word accuracy** (Bradley, Allen, & Clifford, 1983; Schmidt, Howard, & Schmidt, 1983), rather than correct productions of individual target phonemes within words, is calculated by counting only words in which all phonemes are produced correctly and then dividing by the total number of words.

In Phase Three, **Maintenance** is monitored in two steps: conversation outside the session and over time. (See Bradley, 1989, for more details on the application of this program.)

The goal of the Multiple Phonemic program is to be more efficient; however, working on so many targets at the same time can confuse children who have many speech sound deficiencies. Careful data collection and organization of data can be difficult with a large number of clients. SLPs often modify this program by using several, rather than all, phoneme targets.

Linguistic-Based Approaches

How Are Distinctive Features Incorporated in Intervention?

The linguistic theory of distinctive features (Chomsky & Halle, 1968; Jakobson, Fant, & Halle, 1952) is discussed in Chapter 9. The Distinctive Features Approach is based on this, which is a classification system that uses certain features to distinguish phonemes from one another across languages.

The features include consideration of the place and manner of articulation and whether the phoneme is voiced or not. (See Chapter 2 for additional information.) Although there are phonemes that share some features, each is distinct because of at least one differing feature.

Clinical application has generally been experimental and limited. Blache (1978) proposed using this theory to correct speech sound errors; thus features, rather than phonemes, were targeted. Phonemes are classified according to presence/absence of six distinctive features: nasality, voicing, front production, back production, continuation, and stridency. Following classification, a speaker might be described as "lacking a feature" and the objective would develop that feature. Thus, /t/ substituted for /s/ lacks both [+ continuant] and [+ strident]. One or both of these features, rather than individual phoneme production, becomes the target. Subsequent substitutions that included [+ continuant] (e.g., /ʃ/) are reinforced and viewed as progression toward a correct production. In this example, the [+ continuant] feature is demonstrated, along with the extra feature [+ high], which would need to be eliminated before /s/ is produced correctly. Blache did not use production of the isolated phoneme, because he felt that there was an abnormal lengthening of the articulatory gesture in isolation. Instead he used **minimal pairs** (or minimal word pairs). In a minimal word pair, one word in the pair contains the feature and the other does not (e.g., *sea* [+ continuant] and *tea* [– continuant]).

According to McReynolds and Bennett (1972), changes in a feature of one phoneme should generalize to other phonemes that share the same feature. Correct production of phonemes in the same sound class (e.g., strident), especially those with two or more common features (e.g., /s/ and /ʃ/), are more likely to generalize.

Distinctive features were helpful in classifying and understanding the relationship between phonemes. This analysis, however, did not account for phoneme omissions. The classification was not intended to be an intervention approach. Some distinctive feature terms continue to be used (e.g., continuant, strident), although distinctive feature analysis has generally been subsumed under phonological analysis.

What Is the Goal of Phonologically Based Approaches?

Other linguistic-based approaches recognize phonology as a part of the child's communicative system (Hodson & Paden, 1983, 1991; Stoel-Gammon & Dunn,

1985). Although the overall goal of any intervention approach is improving accuracy of speech sound production and increasing intelligibility, an additional goal basic to all phonological intervention is facilitating the reorganization of a child's phonological system and enhancing strategies for processing phonological information (Grunwell, 1985). Objectives for early phonological approaches focused on suppression of "processes" (e.g., suppress fronting) through intervention of sounds (e.g., /k/) affected by the process (Edwards, 1992). (See Chapter 9 for additional information.) The sound system of a language also includes an awareness of patterns. Approaches that develop awareness of patterns include the Cycles Approach (Hodson & Paden, 1991), the Metaphon Approach (Howell & Dean, 1994), and Phonological Awareness Approaches (e.g., Gillon, 2000a).

What Is Targeted in the Cycles Approach?

The Cycles Phonological Remediation Approach (Hodson & Paden, 1991) represents a paradigm shift. It was designed for intervention of highly unintelligible children. The focus is on facilitating the emergence of phonological patterns, contrasted with meeting a criterion for mastery of individual phonemes. In each intervention cycle, several deficient, but stimulable, phonological patterns (e.g., syllableness, /s/ clusters) are targeted, rather than treating individual phonemes in a hierarchy (e.g., word level, sentence level, conversation). According to Hodson and Paden, a Cycles Approach more closely matches the natural acquisition of a child's sound system.

Phonological pattern assessment (e.g., Hodson Assessment of Phonological Patterns–3, Hodson, 2004) yields error patterns of omissions (e.g., consonant sequence reduction, [tɑp] for *stop)* and consonant category deficiencies (e.g., velar deficiencies, [tɑr] for *car).* A phoneme that represents a deficient pattern becomes the target (e.g., /k/ in word-final position for the velar pattern during the first week) for an intervention session (1 hour or 2 half-hour sessions). NOTE: Each week, a different phoneme or word position is targeted, until all stimulable primary patterns have been targeted. The objective is facilitation of the pattern, rather than meeting a set criterion before going on to another target pattern. When a child begins using a target pattern correctly in one word position (e.g., velar in final position), that pattern is not recycled, because this indicates that the target is emerging. (See Chapter 6 for further explanation and Chapter 7 for an example of the Cycles Approach.)

How Is the Metaphon Approach Used to Develop Reorganization of the Sound System?

The Metaphon Approach, a cognitive-linguistic approach, was developed to facilitate cognitive reorganization of children's speech sound systems (Howell & Dean, 1994). The premise is that children can change their sound productions through developing an awareness of the similarities and differences in duration, placement, and manner of production for speech sounds. This awareness is demonstrated through classification sorting.

Metaphon has two phases. In Phase One, phonological production concepts and terminology (e.g., noisy or whispered, front or back) are enhanced through classification (sorting) of nonspeech sounds. In Phase Two, judgment of minimal pair words assists transfer of this knowledge to communication. Children learn to monitor themselves in sentence production and modify what they say for more effective communication. Emphasis on classification activities, rather than production, assists cognitive-linguistic reorganization. Results of a study of Scottish preschoolers (Dean, Howell, Walters, & Reid, 1995) demonstrated that children using this approach improved expressive phonological productions. (See Dean et al. for additional information and applications of the Metaphon Approach.)

How Does Phonological Awareness Influence Expressive Phonology?

Children with expressive phonological impairments, especially children with severe impairments, have been shown to be at greater risk for later literacy problems (Hodson & Strattman, 2004). Results of several studies indicate that there is a relationship between expressive phonological abilities and phonological awareness skills (Bird, Bishop, & Freeman, 1995; Clarke-Klein & Hodson, 1995; Webster & Plante, 1995). Phonological awareness abilities, which include the awareness of the sound structure of a language and the ability to manipulate sounds in words, are highly correlated with literacy success (see Hodson & Strattman, 2004).

Additional studies have shown that phonological awareness can be taught (e.g., Blachman, Ball, Black, & Tangel, 1994). A few intervention studies have reported changes in both phonological awareness and expressive phonology.

Gillon (2000a) found that both expressive phonological productions and phonological awareness skills improved following intervention emphasizing phonological awareness activities. (See Chapter 8 for additional information.)

How Can a Whole Language Approach Affect Expressive Phonology?

Children with expressive phonological deviations often have other language impairments. Language-based intervention (Hoffman, Norris, & Monjure, 1990; Norris & Hoffman, 1990; Tyler, Lewis, Haskill, & Tolbert, 2002) has been utilized to facilitate improvement of all aspects of language in more natural communication situations. In particular, these approaches address language use beyond the word level.

Hoffman et al. espoused "whole to part" learning by using interactive storytelling to facilitate phonological development and improve semantic and syntactic skills. As the children talked about action-oriented pictures, the SLP provided scaffolding for the children's narratives, encouraging them to (1) clarify deficient sound productions, sentence structure, or semantic relationships; (2) add information; and (3) increase the complexity by including relationships (e.g., cause-effect) and motivation (e.g., feelings). The SLP modeled the enhanced language, and children were given opportunities to restate. Results of this approach were efficient and effective for children with mild impairment. Other studies, however, have shown that children with more severe phonological deficiencies may need more direct phonological intervention (Fey, 1992; Tyler et al., 2002).

Target Selection Considerations

Choosing remediation targets is extremely important, especially for children who are unintelligible. Although targets for phoneme-oriented approaches have been selected based on a variety of factors, choosing appropriate remediation targets is a primary focal point for current intervention approaches. Minimal pair contrasts are used in some approaches, whereas targets for other approaches are maximal contrasts. In some approaches, stimulability is a prerequisite, while other approaches recommend targets of least phonological ability. Choosing target phonemes within the child's **zone of proximal development** (Vygotsky, 1978) has been found to be "what the child is ready to learn with some help from a competent adult" (Paul, 2001, p. 65). The zone of proximal development refers to what the child currently does independently and his or her potential with adequate support. In the next section, targets for phoneme-oriented approaches, contrast approaches, and pattern-oriented approaches will be discussed.

Targets for Phoneme-Oriented Approaches

How Are Target Phonemes Selected?

In most phoneme-oriented approaches, phoneme errors are determined by using a standardized articulation test. Errors of **substitutions, omissions, distortions,** and/or **additions (SODA)** are tallied (Van Riper, 1939). Generally, errors are identified in single, one- or two-syllable words that have phonemes in the initial, medial, or final position in the word (e.g., /s/ in *sun, dresser, bus).* The other phonemes in the target word typically are not assessed. One or two (the voiced or voiceless cognate) target phonemes are chosen for intervention. The selection for phoneme-oriented intervention are based on one or more of the following factors:

- **Chronological or developmental age of the child.** Standardized tests and sound development scales (e.g., Prather, Hendrick, & Kern, 1975; Smit, Hand, Freilinger, Bernthal, & Bird, 1990; Templin, 1957) are used to identify earliest developing phonemes, which are targeted first (see Chapter 3). Although there are numerous differences among development scales, early developing phonemes are considered a prerequisite for acquiring later developing phonemes.
- **Phoneme frequency.** Correct production of phonemes used frequently in the language can increase intelligibility (e.g., /s/ is a frequently occurring phoneme, as well as a morphological marker for plurality, possession, and third-person singular verbs).
- **Stimulability.** The ability to **imitate** a sound after a model or placement instructions facilitates remediation progress. Sounds that are stimulable are chosen before sounds that are not stimulable.

- **Visibility.** Phonemes that children can easily observe being produced by looking in a mirror may be targets. For example, placement of the bottom lip on the central incisors for production of /f/ is one of the most visible.
- **Variability inconsistency.** Sounds that are produced intermittently (correctly in some words or phonetic contexts) may suggest that children are "working" internally on these sounds.
- **Utility.** Family members may request, or a clinician may choose, a target based on utility at home or school (e.g., first sound in the child's, sibling's, or pet's name).

The goal of phoneme-oriented approaches is correct production of individual phonemes in natural-speaking situations (carryover). An additional goal is generalization to untreated phonemes that share manner of production, placement, or voicing, although this is not assured.

Another point of view is to target phonemes that represent "least productive phonological knowledge" (Elbert, 1992; Gierut, Morrisette, Hughes, & Rowland, 1996). Two or more phonemes that are neither stimulable nor early developing are selected. The phonemes selected represent inventory constraints or phonemes or features that are not present in any position. Based on a series of single-subject design studies, Gierut et al. recommended least phonological knowledge targets to increase generalization potential. Rvachew and Nowak (2001) challenged their recommendation based on results of a randomized-control study. Results were poorer for the children who targeted nonstimulable least phonological knowledge first.

Targets for Contrast Approaches

Speech sound intervention using contrasting pairs of words has been recommended for many years (Fairbanks, 1960). Approaches that use contrasting words as targets include Minimal Pairs, Maximal Oppositions, and Multiple Oppositions.

What Is the Target Focus of Minimal Pairs?

Minimal Pair contrasts have been used to demonstrate to children with phoneme substitutions (e.g., [t] for /k/) that substituting a different phoneme (e.g., [tep] for *cape),* creates another word that means something different. These words differ minimally, by one phoneme. Distinctive feature research and intervention (e.g., Blache, 1978; Costello & Onstine, 1976; McReynolds & Bennett, 1972) use minimal word pairs. A feature was taught using a word with and without the target feature (e.g., *tea* and *sea* for [– continuant and + continuant]).

Blache (1978) advocated using a Montessori-based "discovery" concept with Minimal Pair words. Children discover a need to produce a particular phoneme because another sound created a different word. Different phonemes were required to distinguish between the two, usually pictured on separate cards (e.g., *tail* and *sail).*

Weiner reported a similar method with Minimal Pair Contrasts (Weiner, 1981). Children played a game that required selection of an appropriate picture (a *boat* but not a *bow)* from an array. Failure to produce the target word created misunderstanding and resulted in a breakdown of communication.

What Is the Target Focus of Maximal Oppositions?

In the early research with Maximal Opposition targets, Elbert and Gierut (1986) and Gierut (2001) contrasted phonemes that differed widely, often involving three or more distinctive features. For Maximal Oppositions, the number of distinctive feature differences is calculated. Although there are major distinctive feature differences (vocalic and sonorant) between /l/ and /k/, two phonemes a young child is often missing from his or her inventory, only the seven nonmajor differences (high, back, lateral, interrupted, coronal, continuant, and voiced) are counted. There is maximal opposition between /l/ and /k/ because of the number of feature differences. Gierut (1992) contrasted two sounds not in the child's inventory, phonemes that differed most and by major class features. In her research, children had at least six sounds missing in their phonetic and phonemic inventories. Based on case study findings, Gierut advocated using this method for children with moderate to severe phonological disorders. (See Gierut, 2001, for additional information.) Children with severe deviations, who cannot produce either of these phonemes, would have difficulty reaching the set criterion. This presents a mismatch with the zone of proximal development, as well as early success in intervention (e.g., Van Riper & Emerick, 1984; McCabe & Bradley, 1975). In addition, Fey (1992) commented that activities for maximal contrasts are "more limited to contrived [rather than natural] intervention activities than minimal pair procedure" (p. 280).

What Is the Target Focus of Multiple Oppositions?

Single phoneme targets are contrasted in both Minimal Pair and Maximal Opposition Approaches. In the Multiple Oppositions Approach (Williams, 2000b), several targets are contrasted simultaneously with the child's substitution (e.g., [ti] for *key, sea,* and *she).* Williams (2000a) designed this approach for the child with severe to profound phonological deviations who substitutes or collapses one phoneme for several, very different phonemes. This **homonymy** likely contributes greatly to reduced intelligibility. The premise is that the child's sound system will be reorganized through experience with several different targets. Intervention phases include (a) imitation, (b) spontaneous phrases, (c) spontaneous contrasts with untrained words, and (d) naturalistic conversation. Although results of Williams's experimental treatment were positive, there are concerns relative to the child's motivation early in intervention and intervention utility. (See Williams, 2000a, 2000b, for the theoretical basis and experimental treatment design.)

Targets for Pattern-Oriented Approaches

How Are Target Patterns Selected?

The sound patterns in a language include not only the phonemes, but also the phoneme production within the word context. Patterns include syllables, consonant word endings and beginnings, and consonant sequences. Omission of any of these patterns may affect intelligibility more than a single phoneme substitution or distortion. Deviations involving consonant categories (e.g., stridents) can be caused by omissions or substitutions of consonants from differing categories. (See Chapter 4 for definitions and examples.) Knowledge of these deviations, beyond phonetic inventories, yields a more complete understanding of a child's phonological system. Target patterns for intervention are based on omissions and consonant category deficiencies that facilitate the reorganization of that system, rather than correcting individual phonemes. Targeting omissions and deviations of early developing patterns increases intelligibility rapidly. More detailed information regarding optimal target patterns is provided in Chapter 6.

Summary

Intervention approaches for speech sound deviations have been influenced by theories that have affected the entire profession. Initially, the emphasis was on correction of individual sounds. Phoneme-oriented approaches were designed to correct "articulation" deviations. Various approaches were used to correct placement, manner, and voicing errors. Phoneme-oriented methods are appropriate for children with mild impairments (e.g., lisps). Behavioristic theories influenced intervention. Linguistic theories broadened the view of speech sound intervention.

Phonological theories have led to the most recent, far-reaching intervention changes—facilitating the reorganization of a child's communication system. Assessment of phonological patterns allows insight into the child's system. The overall goal is intelligibility. Understanding the salient points of intervention approaches and choosing targets according to the unique needs of the child facilitates attainment of that goal.

PART III

Applications for Children with Highly Unintelligible Speech

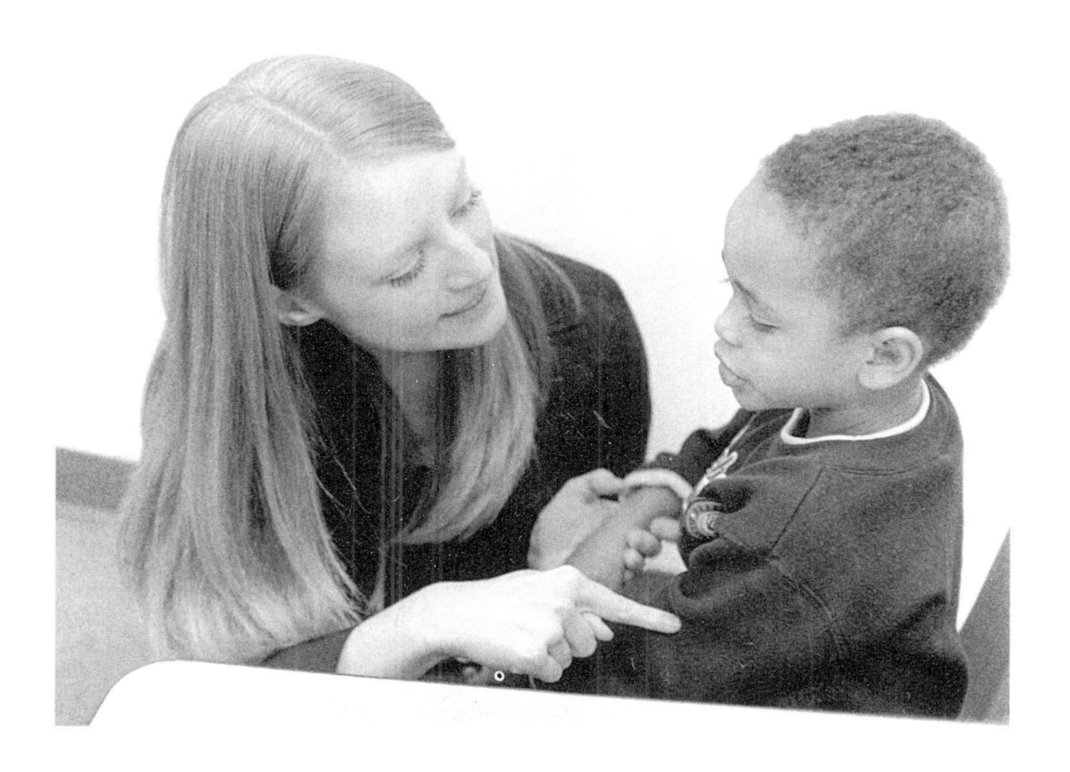

CHAPTER 6

Enhancing Children's Phonological Systems— The Cycles Remediation Approach

Barbara Williams Hodson

Basic Considerations

- What Are Cycles?
- How Are Target Patterns Selected and Presented?

Target Patterns

- What Are Potential Optimal Primary Target Patterns for Beginning Cycles?
- What Are Potential Secondary Target Patterns?
- Which Targets Are Inappropriate for Preschoolers?
- What Are Advanced Target Patterns?

Intervention

- How Are Children Helped to Develop Awareness of Phonological Patterns?
- What Is the General Structure for Phonological Intervention Sessions?
- What Is the "Home" Program?
- How Are Production-Practice Words Selected?
- What Are Typical Production-Practice Activities?
- Why and How Are Phonological Awareness Activities Incorporated?
- When and Why Is Focused Auditory Stimulation Used?

Theoretical & Conceptual Considerations

- What Theoretical/Conceptual Aspects Influenced the Cycles Phonological Remediation Approach?
- What Underlying Concepts Guide the Cycles Approach?
- What Published Evidence Is Available Regarding Effectiveness of Targeting and Cycling Phonological Patterns?

Additional Considerations
Summary

The approach described in this chapter—the Cycles Phonological Remediation Approach—was designed explicitly for children with highly unintelligible speech, including clients with the label of suspected Childhood Apraxia of Speech (see Vellemann, 2003). The primary factor that differentiates the Cycles Phonological Remediation Approach (also referred to simply as the Cycles Approach) from phoneme-oriented programs (described in Chapter 5) is that deficient **phonological patterns** (e.g., final consonants, /s/ clusters) are facilitated in a cyclical fashion to expedite **intelligibility** gains (Hodson, 1978, 1982, 1994a, 1997, 1998, 2005; Hodson & Paden, 1983, 1991). The Cycles Approach evolved as a result of formulating and testing clinical research hypotheses while working with several hundred children between the ages of 2½ and 14 years.

This chapter begins by providing general information about cycles and then optimal target patterns. Intervention is the third major section. The last section includes information about theoretical and conceptual considerations for phonological intervention.

Basic Considerations

What Are Cycles?

A **cycle,** which is a period of time, is completed only after all of the phonological patterns that need to be targeted (including liquids, if deficient) have been presented. The length of each cycle depends on the number of deficient patterns an individual child has, as well as the number of deficient sounds that are **stimulable** (i.e., consonants a child is not producing but can imitate or produce with assists) within each of the patterns. Some cycles extend for 5 or 6 weeks (typically 1 contact hour per week) in length; others may be as long as 15 or 16 weeks.

Phonemes within targeted patterns are used to facilitate emergence of the respective phonological patterns. In other words, phonemes serve as a "means to an end" rather than an "end in themselves." Each phonological pattern (e.g., /s/ clusters) is targeted for 2 to 6 hours per cycle; each target phoneme (or consonant cluster; e.g., word-initial /sp/) within the pattern is facilitated for approximately 60 minutes. The first cycle lays a **phonological foundation** and allows children to experience early success on target patterns in carefully selected production-practice words. Generalization to conversation is not expected until the second or third cycle.

Phonological patterns are **recycled** (i.e., re-presented) during ensuing cycles until they begin to emerge in spontaneous conversational utterances. **Complexity** is increased gradually during succeeding cycles by incorporating production-practice words with more difficult phonetic environments (see Kent, 1982) and also by grouping phonemes within target patterns (e.g., /sp/ and /st/ re-presented together during a second-cycle session).

How Are Target Patterns Selected and Presented?

Each child's phonological system is evaluated first (see Chapter 4) to determine if any of the potential primary target patterns are deficient (see Table 6.1, page 90). Secondary patterns (see Table 6.2, page 97) are not targeted until certain criteria are met. Advanced patterns are targeted by individuals above the age of 8 years with "intelligibility" issues who experience difficulty producing complex multisyllabic words.

A highly unintelligible client's phonological intervention begins with facilitation of a pattern for which **readiness** is demonstrated. This does not mean that it is appropriate, however, to target phonemes that the child already produces (even if inconsistent). Rather, the most stimulable pattern from the client's **phonological deficiencies** is selected for enhancement so that the child can experience immediate and tangible success (Hunt, 1961). The second most stimulable pattern is targeted next, and so on until all deficient primary patterns are facilitated during each cycle.

The specific patterns/phonemes and the order of presentation within a cycle depend, of course, on each individual child's phonological abilities. Target patterns that have not yet begun to emerge in conversational speech by the beginning of each ensuing cycle are recycled.

Each phoneme (or consonant cluster) within a pattern is targeted for approximately 60 minutes per cycle (i.e., one 60-minute, two 30-minute, or three 20-minute sessions) before progressing to the next phoneme in that pattern and then on to other deficient phonological patterns. Furthermore, it is desirable to provide stimulation for two or more target phonemes (in successive weeks) within a pattern before changing to the next target pattern (i.e., each deficient phonological pattern is stimulated for 2 hours or more within each cycle). Only one phonological pattern is targeted during a beginning cycles session, allowing the child to

Table 6.1 *Potential Primary Target Patterns for Beginning Cycles*

Word Structures/Phonotactics
Syllableness (for omitted vowels, diphthongs, vocalic/syllabic consonants resulting in productions limited to monosyllables)
• 2-syllable compound words (e.g., *cowboy, ice cream)* for appropriate number of syllables • 3-syllable/word combinations (e.g., *cowboy hat, ice-cream cone)*
Singleton Consonants (when consistently omitted per word positions below)
• Prevocalic consonants; **CV** (word-initial /p/, /b/, /m/, /w/) • Postvocalic consonants; **VC** (voiceless final stops /p, t, k/; possibly final /m/, /n/) • Pre- and postvocalic consonants; **CVC** (e.g., *pup, pop)* • Intervocalic consonants; **VCV** (e.g., *apple)*
/s/ Clusters
• Word-initial (e.g., /sp/, /st/) • Word-final (e.g., /ts/, /ps/)
Anterior/Posterior Contrasts
• Word-final /k/ • Word-initial /k/, /g/ (for "fronters") • Occasionally /h/ • Alveolars/Labials (if "backer")
Liquids
• Word-initial /l/ • Word-initial /r/ (suppress gliding initially) • Word-initial /kr/, /gr/ (after the child readily produces singleton velars) • Word-initial /l/ clusters (after child readily produces prevocalic /l/)

Source: Hodson (1997)

focus. Patterns are not intermingled (e.g., final /k/ in the same session as initial /st/) until the third or fourth cycle.

Target Patterns

What Are Potential Optimal Primary Target Patterns for Beginning Cycles?

Word Structures (Omissions)

Most 2-year-olds with typical development produce word-initial singleton stops, nasals, and glides (particularly labials) and some word-final nasals and voiceless obstruents (Preisser, Hodson, & Paden, 1988; Stoel-Gammon & Dunn, 1985). Furthermore, 2-year-olds commonly produce utterances that contain two or three syllables, as well as word-initial and word-final consonants. Children with expressive phonological impairments vary greatly in their abilities to produce these early developing phoneme classes (i.e., stops, nasals, and glides) and word structures ("syllableness," prevocalic/postvocalic/intervocalic singleton consonants).

Syllableness (Omission of the syllable nuclei: vowels, diphthongs, vocalic/syllabic consonants)

Most preschool children sequence at least two syllables (e.g., *Mama).* For clients who have not yet learned to produce syllables in sequences, two- and three-syllable compound words (e.g., *cowboy, ice-cream cone)* are optimal early targets. The emphasis during this time is on the appropriate number of syllables (i.e., vowels, diphthongs, vocalic/syllabic phonemes) rather than on the accuracy of specific consonants. After children learn to sequence two and three syllables, most will begin to produce two- and three-word phrases or sentences in their spontaneous conversational speech, within a few weeks.

Singleton Consonants

The **C**V syllable structure (i.e., word-initial singleton consonant) does not often need to be targeted. Most children produce some initial consonants, but the repertoire may be restricted (e.g., all stops). When a child consistently deletes word-initial consonants, the labial stops /p, b/, nasal /m/, and glide /w/ can be presented to help the individual learn to produce prevocalic consonants.

Omissions of word-final singletons (**VC**) are fairly common in utterances of children with intelligibility issues. This phenomenon is sometimes referred to as open syllable, final consonant deletion, or CV (consonant vowel) preference. Children with highly unintelligible speech delete word-final obstruents more often than word-final nasals. Postvocalic voiceless stops (/p/, /t/, and/or /k/, depending on stimulability) and/or anterior nasals (word-final /m, n/, if lacking) are appropriate phoneme targets to help children develop their abilities to close syllables.

Occasionally a child produces final consonants in some words and initial consonants in others, but fails to produce **CVC** (initial and final consonants in the same word). Monosyllabic words containing the same initial and final consonant (e.g., *pipe, mom)* help children to produce both consonants and to learn that consonants can occur at the beginning and also the end of the same word. Some children produce word-initial and word-final consonants, but delete medial consonants V**C**V. In such instances, two-syllable words with medial stop consonants (e.g., *apple)* are useful to help children begin producing intervocalic consonants.

/s/ Clusters

Every highly unintelligible client (school-age, as well as preschool) who participated in the university phonology clinics evidenced consonant sequence/cluster reductions. Preschool clients commonly delete stridency either by substitution (e.g., [ti] for *sea;* [poɚ] for *four)* or omission (e.g., [pɑt] for *spot;* [no] for *nose).*

Highly unintelligible school-age clients often produce singleton stridents (especially if they have already participated in phoneme-oriented singleton /s/ intervention programs) but still experience great difficulty producing /s/ clusters/sequences. These school-age clients typically produce the /s/, but delete other consonant(s) in the sequence (e.g., [sɪk] for *stick).* Teaching children to produce /s/ clusters at an early age increases **intelligibility** quickly and also seems to have far-reaching effects. Moreover, the emergence of /s/ clusters serves to reduce two major deviations—strident category deficiency and consonant sequence reduction.

For children who substitute stops for strident phonemes, /s/ is targeted first in words containing /s/ clusters (e.g., *stand)* rather than as a singleton (e.g., *sand).* The primary reason for this is because it has been observed repeatedly that when clinicians attempt to elicit singleton /s/ first, clients with highly unintelligible speech typically produce /s/ plus stop combinations (e.g., [sti] for *see).* It is easier initially for these children to produce words with /s/ clusters rather than singleton /s/. Moreover, most preschool children will then generalize to /s/ singleton without it ever actually being targeted.

Another consideration is that an emphasis on prevocalic singleton /s/ sometimes has created two additional problems for highly unintelligible clients. Children who have been taught to say singleton /s/ and to suppress their inclination to produce an intervening stop have typically experienced difficulty later when they attempt to produce /s/ clusters (e.g., /s_ɑp/ for *stop).* A second problem that has commonly co-occurred has been a distortion of /s/. A number of clients who already had received singleton /s/ programming tended to palatalize or lateralize /s/. It is likely that their clinicians had modeled an exaggerated /s/, with a common outcome being distorted sibilant productions.

The actual selection order for /s/ cluster targets depends on each client's phonological system. For example, for a child who demonstrates velar fronting, initial /sk/ (e.g., *sky)* or final /ks/ (e.g., *rocks)* should **not** be targeted during beginning cycles (i.e., only after facility in producing singleton velars is demonstrated). Likewise, for a child who demonstrates backing of alveolar stops, /st/ or /ts/ should not be targeted until alveolars have begun to emerge, or /sp/ or /ps/ if labials are lacking. Moreover, for a child who lacks nasals, /sm/ or /sn/ should not be targeted until the child produces nasals spontaneously.

Although word-final and word-initial /s/ clusters are both targeted during each of the first few cycles, they are not intermingled until later cycles. Thus stimulable word-initial /s/ clusters (/sp/, /sm/, /sn/, /st/, and/or /sk/, and occasionally /sw/ and /sl/) are targeted in succession, then set aside until the next cycle, before (or after) targeting stimulable word-final /s/ clusters (/ts/, /ps/, and/or /ks/).

A carrier phrase (*It's a ______)* is usually incorporated with practice words containing /s/ clusters by the third cycle (after a child demonstrates facility producing /s/ clusters in monosyllabic production-practice words). During one session, the child uses the carrier phrase for words that do not contain /s/ (e.g., *It's a door).* The next session the child is taught how to produce an /s/-cluster word in the *It's a* _____ phrase (e.g., *It's a star).* The purpose for this task is to have the child produce /s/ twice in an utterance (in the correct positions in the phrase), rather than for practice in phrases/sentences. Typically, stridency begins emerging in spontaneous utterances 5 or 6 weeks after the child experiences success with this task. (NOTE: This is the only "phrase" work that is incorporated in intervention sessions for preschool children.)

Anterior/Posterior Contrasts

When children lack velars or alveolars because of omissions and/or fronting (e.g., [ti] for *key)* or backing (e.g., [ki] for *tea),* anterior/posterior contrasts are targeted. Word-final /k/ and then word-initial /g/ and/or /k/ (without concern regarding voicing) are targeted (if stimulable) when a child lacks velars. Children who are "backers" typically need to target alveolar stops (i.e., /t, d/), but occasionally labials need to be targeted. The selection, of course, depends on which pattern is deficient, as well as which phonemes are stimulable.

Velars need to be targeted considerably more often than alveolars. Many children have extreme difficulty producing /k/ during the first cycle. It may be necessary in such instances to delay production-practice activities on velar phonemes for several months until the child is stimulable for a velar. During this period, efforts should be made during each session to **stimulate** velar production. Assists such as tactile cues and amplification often are effective. One technique that has been useful for some children has been for the clinician to model the voiceless velar fricative /x/, rather than the velar stop /k/. After the child develops the kinesthetic image for the /x/, it is relatively easy to move to production of the velar stop /k/ counterpart.

The glottal fricative /h/ is another posterior phoneme that some children need to target. In our clinic, we have found, however, that simply showing a child how to produce /h/ often suffices without actually targeting /h/ directly. (NOTE: In some instances, posterior consonants are targeted before /s/ clusters when velars are stimulable.)

Liquids

The /l/ and /r/ phonemes (if lacking) are stimulated/facilitated, as well, at the end of each cycle. Although liquid gliding is still relatively common in utterances of 4-year-olds with typical development (Grunwell, 1987; Hodson & Paden, 1981), approximately half of the children in developmental phonology studies (e.g., Dyson, 1988; Porter & Hodson, 2001) produced liquids appropriately by age 3.

Moreover, it is of some interest to note that a surprising number of highly unintelligible 3- and 4-year-old clients who had extremely limited speech-sound repertoires demonstrated excellent word-final vocalic /ɚ, ɝ/ productions during their initial assessment sessions.

Another clinical observation has been that if liquids were targeted only after all other phonological patterns were established, children typically required several additional years of intervention in order to develop their abilities to produce liquids (particularly /r/). Clinical records indicate that when stimulation for liquids was provided at the end of every cycle, clients demonstrated closer approximations of liquids during each ensuing cycle. Furthermore, some spontaneous liquid productions began to emerge during the periods that other targeted patterns (e.g., velars, /s/ clusters) were being generalized into conversation. Target words for liquids should be chosen with extreme care. Words with labial consonants /p, b, m, w, f, v/ (e.g., *leaf)* and/or round vowels /u, o/ (e.g., *row)* must be avoided during early cycles because of potential labial assimilation effects that encourage productions of /w/ rather than /r/ or /l/.

Typically, the client is taught to click his or her tongue tip (independent of jaw movement) the week before /l/ is targeted. Caregivers are encouraged to have the child practice the tongue-tip clicking activity every day for one week. If the child does this task, it usually is relatively easy to elicit appropriate productions of /l/ in carefully selected practice words during the ensuing session.

When targeting word-initial /r/, blending is de-emphasized during the first couple of cycles (in order to suppress insertion of /w/), and the vowel following /r/ is prolonged and exaggerated. Thus, for the target word *rock,* the clinician models /ɝ/ (with jaw lowered and mouth in a wide open position), then pauses, and then says /ɑ:k/ (prolonging the vowel and often altering the pitch). The client must not be allowed to insert /w/. At first, most children say /ʊ/ rather than /ɝ/, which is accepted during the beginning cycles as long as the client does not insert /w/. (NOTE: Prevocalic /r/ is presented at the end of each cycle even if the child is not actually stimulable for an accurate /r/ production. We have observed that children demonstrate closer approximations of /r/ during each succeeding cycle.)

Velar-liquid clusters /kl, gl, kr, gr/ usually are targeted by the third or fourth cycle (provided the child has developed facility in producing /k/ and /g/). When velar /r/ clusters are presented, the clinician emphasizes the vocalic /ɝ/ and then pauses before producing and prolonging the vowel (e.g., /kɝ aɪ/ for *cry).* For velar /l/ clusters, a schwa is inserted initially for the model (e.g., /kəlɑk/ for *clock).* The schwa is "faded" as the child gains facility producing /l/ in clusters.

Alveolar-liquid clusters /tr, dr, sl/ can be presented, as well, during recycling of liquid clusters. Labial liquid clusters /pl, bl, fl, pr, br, fr/ should be the last liquid clusters to be targeted because of possible labial assimilation effects related to the labial consonants /p, b, f/.

School-age clients often need to target postvocalic /ɚ, ɝ/ and word-medial /l/ and /r/ consonants. Most preschool clients who have developed a good phonological foundation, however, demonstrate liquid generalization to other word positions without direct intervention.

What Are Potential Secondary Target Patterns?

Potential secondary patterns (see Table 6.2) are not targeted until after specific criteria have been met. The following patterns must have been acquired in spontaneous utterances (1) **syllableness;** (2) basic word structures (i.e., no omissions of singleton consonants)**;** and (3) **anterior/posterior contrasts,** although some assimilations (e.g., *goggie* for *doggie)* may still occur. Moreover, clients also must evidence emergence of **stridency** in their conversations and **suppression** of the glide substitution/insertion for production-practice words that contain **liquids.**

Most secondary patterns will no longer be problematic after cycles for the primary patterns have been completed. Typically these patterns emerge while children are working on the primary patterns. This is particularly true for preschool clients who seem to develop other components of their phonological systems and who generalize exceptionally well during the time they are improving their listening skills and learning to produce the primary patterns. Using **minimal-pair** words that contrast the child's actual erroneous productions (e.g., contrasting *let* with *yet* rather than *wet* for the child who substitutes /j/ for /l/) is extremely helpful when targeting secondary patterns to facilitate understanding of the semantic difference(s) between target words and error production.

If reassessment following the cycle in which the above criteria are met indicates that any secondary patterns are still deficient, these patterns become targets

Table 6.2 *Potential Secondary Target Patterns*

(Target only those that remain problematic. Incorporate minimal pairs whenever possible.)

Palatals
• Glide /j/ • Palatal sibilants /ʃ, ʒ, ʧ, ʤ/ • Vocalic /ɚ/, /ɝ/ (unless dialectal) • Word-medial /r/
Other Consonant Sequences
• Word-medial and word-final /s/ plus stop (e.g., *basket, desk)* • CC with sonorants
• Glide clusters (e.g., /kw, kj/)   • Other liquid clusters (e.g., /tr/)
• **CCC** (e.g., /skw, skr/
Singleton Stridents (e.g., /f, s/)
Voicing Contrasts (Prevocalic only)
Vowel Contrasts (Nondialectal)
Assimilations
Any Remaining Idiosyncratic Deviations

Source: Hodson (1997)

for final cycles. **Prevocalic voicing** (e.g., *do* for *to),* **vowel neutralization** (e.g., *hut* for *hat*, *hit*, etc.), **assimilations** (e.g., *numb* for *thumb),* and/or **idiosyncratic phonological rules** (Fey & Gandour, 1982; Leonard, Schwartz, Swanson, & Frome-Loeb, 1987) rarely need to be targeted, however, even though they may have been prevalent at the onset of intervention.

Singleton **stridents** may be targeted, if still problematic, after /s/ clusters are emerging in conversation. Preschool clients typically demonstrate generalization to singleton strident phonemes (particularly /f/ and /s/) after targeting /s/ clusters for a couple of cycles. If a child still inserts a stop, the procedure of exaggerating or prolonging the vowel, rather than prolonging the initial consonant (e.g., /si:/ rather than /s:i/ for *sea),* also helps the child learn to produce words containing singleton stridents without inserting the intervening stop consonant.

Palatal phonemes may still be problematic for children at this time. Some clients need to target palatal sibilants because of depalatalization (e.g.,

[su] for *shoe)* and/or affrication (e.g., [ʧu] for *shoe)* or deaffrication (e.g., [ʃer] for *chair),* but palatal sibilants are not targeted until the final cycles, and then only if they have not yet begun to emerge in the child's conversational speech. If a child does not yet produce the palatal glide, /j/ should be taught before targeting palatal sibilants. For children who evidence depalatalization, the combination of the sibilant followed by the palatal glide /j/ is modeled initially (e.g., [sju] for *shoe,* [tsju] for *chew).* After the child develops the new kinesthetic image for palatal sibilants, coalescence yields the actual palatal sibilant. An example of this phenomenon is the common production by American-English speakers of /mɪʃu/ for *miss you.* The other palatal sound that commonly needs facilitation at this time is the liquid, particularly vocalic /ɚ, ɝ/. In addition, /r/ may need to be targeted in other consonant clusters and in word-medial position.

Any remaining deficient **consonant sequences** are targeted during final phonological cycles. Clusters containing glides (e.g., /kw, tw, sw, bj, fj, hj, kj, mj/) are troublesome for some clients, as are certain medial and final consonant clusters. Some clients demonstrate excessive difficulty producing medial /s/ clusters (e.g., *biscuit, boxing)* and final /s/ clusters with the /s/ preceding the stop (e.g., *desk, toast).* Medial and final /s/ + stop clusters and three-consonant clusters (e.g., *string, mixed)* are common targets during the final cycles.

One of the salient clinical research findings over the years has been that targeting consonant clusters (particularly /s/ clusters) is of the utmost importance (Hodson & Paden, 1991). Children who are less intelligible in conversational speech than when naming single words usually are experiencing difficulty producing consonants in sequences that cross syllable/word boundaries. These children delete word endings more often in connected speech than when naming single words. In most instances, however, such deletions are an artifact of consonant sequence reduction, rather than simply word-final singleton consonant deletions. If one word ends in a consonant and the next word begins with a consonant, children who experience difficulty producing two contiguous consonants typically delete one of the consonants, particularly if an /s/ is involved (e.g., "ni puppy" for *nice puppy).*

Which Targets Are Inappropriate for Preschoolers?

Findings from developmental phonology studies (e.g., Porter & Hodson, 2001) have helped identify "productions" that are phonologically typical for children and thus are not considered to be appropriate targets for preschool clients. These targets are listed in Table 6.3. Children with typical development usually prolong the preceding vowel slightly, but do not produce fully voiced word-final obstruents (Higgs & Hodson, 1978; Hodson & Paden, 1981). Most 4-year-olds, for example, typically say /peɪ:ʧ/ (with slight vowel prolongation) rather than /peɪʤ/ for *page*. Furthermore, they commonly use slight pitch alterations for vocalic /l/ in words such as *doll, candle,* and *milk,* but do not exhibit tongue-tip elevation to the alveolar ridge for /l/ in such words. Substitutions of /n/ for /ŋ/, particularly in bisyllabic words (e.g., *runnin* for *running),* and /f, v, s, z/ for /θ, ð/, which are common in utterances of young children with typical phonological development, do not affect intelligibility adversely. In addition, weak/unstressed syllable deletion (e.g., "*member*" for *remember; "probly"* for *probably)* is extremely common in conversational utterances of adult speakers, as well. It therefore seems inappropriate to ask preschool children who have intelligibility issues to produce patterns/phonemes that are "superior" to those of their peers with typical phonological development. Voiced final obstruents /b, d, v, g, z, ð, ʒ, ʤ, final /ŋ/, postvocalic/syllabic /l/, "weak syllables" and /θ, ð/ therefore should not be selected as primary targets for young unintelligible clients.

Table 6.3 *Inappropriate Targets for Preschool Clients*

Targets	*Examples*
Voiced Word-Final Obstruents	/b, d, g, v, z, ð, ʒ, ʤ/
Postvocalic/Syllabic /l/	*ball*
Word-Final /ŋ/	*going*
/θ, ð/	*mouth*
Unstressed (Weak) Syllables	*refrigerator*

Source: Hodson (1997)

What Are Advanced Target Patterns?

Some individuals (above the age of 8 years) experience extreme difficulty producing multisyllabic words (e.g., *aluminum, thermometer)* and complex consonant sequences (e.g., /kskj/ and /kstr/, as in *excuse* and *extra).* These children often are able to name words on a standardized "articulation" test without error, but reduced intelligibility is noted in their conversational utterances. Many come from the ranks of students with language/learning disorders. Some may be former phonology clients who were dismissed because they had become intelligible and had age-appropriate speech at that time.

Clinicians, teachers, and caregivers are asked to develop lists of troublesome words that the student needs to be able to say. Analysis and synthesis techniques for producing such words can be taught, and opportunities for practicing parts and then wholes can be provided. First, the student is taught how to break troublesome words into syllables. Then "phonic writing" is used to determine the specific sounds in each syllable. The next step involves practice in producing all of the sounds in each syllable. Then production combining two syllables is practiced, followed by three syllables, and so on, until the student is able to produce the whole word correctly. Then sentences are generated using the new productions of words to facilitate automaticity and carryover.

Intervention

How Are Children Helped to Develop Awareness of Phonological Patterns?

The purpose of production practice is not to establish a motor pattern. Rather, producing targets in a limited number of carefully selected words provides opportunities for developing new, accurate **kinesthetic** images and for **integrative rehearsal.** It is imperative, as well, to help the child develop **auditory awareness** of the pattern. Unintelligible children do not seem to "hear" their own errors. For example, when adults repeat a word exactly as it was said by a child, the typical response by that child is tell the adult, "no," and then repeat the word with the identical error (Berko & Brown, 1960).

Unintelligible children seem to rely solely on their own inaccurate kinesthetic images that "feel right" at the time and tend to ignore or negate auditory feedback for their inaccurate productions. Combining a limited amount of production practice with slightly amplified auditory stimulation (Clifton & Elliott, 1982; Van Riper, 1939) during each session helps children improve their **phonological representations** of articulatory **gestures** and, ultimately, their **self-monitoring** skills. An amplifier is used whenever a client experiences special difficulty during attempts to produce a particular word.

It must be emphasized that this remediation approach should not be used without incorporating slight amplification, particularly during the first few cycles. Children respond differently when the listening list is presented with amplification than when the practitioner simply says the words loudly. One problem that often accompanies the recitation of words without amplification is that practitioners tend to exaggerate their models, particularly for /s/. It is imperative that a soft, precise /s/ be modeled. Young children tend to "overproduce" what has been modeled, with the common result being distorted sibilants. Moreover, a precise /s/ production seems to enable the child to experience more definitive kinesthetic image feedback.

Traditional visual and tactile cues are incorporated as supplements when needed. For example, when /s/ clusters are introduced, we typically slide a finger (on the child's arm) while saying /s/ and then tap the arm for the second consonant. In many instances, clients temporarily use this tactile cue themselves during the first cycle. These cues are "faded" as the child demonstrates facility producing the target phonemes.

What Is the General Structure for Phonological Intervention Sessions?

The following format has been used in university phonology clinics. This format also has been adapted and used effectively in schools, clinics, and hospitals.

1. The child reviews the preceding session's production-practice word cards. (NOTE: If this is the very first session and there are no prior production-practice cards, the 12-word screening instrument from the *Hodson Assessment of Phonological Patterns* (HAPP–3; 2004) is administered first.) If target patterns are being changed (e.g., velars last session; /s/ clusters this session), the cards from the preceding session are then filed away until a later cycle. They can be reused, and new

words with more difficult phonetic environments can be added during ensuing cycles to increase complexity. If the phoneme target for this session is within the same target pattern as during the preceding session (e.g., /s/ clusters for both sessions), both sets of cards (e.g., /sp/ words from last session and /st/ words for this session) are incorporated into some of the production-practice activities for the current session.

2. The clinician provides slightly amplified **auditory stimulation** of the session's target pattern for about 30 seconds. The child listens while the clinician reads the session's listening list of approximately 20 words that contain the target pattern. (The child is not to repeat these words; rather he or she listens attentively while the clinician reads the list fairly quickly.) The words on this listening list do not need to be selected carefully for phonetic environment considerations. Sometimes the error production is contrasted with the target pattern. At the end of the amplified listening activity, while still wearing the amplifier's headset, the child says some words into the microphone from a second list that contains potential production-practice words.

3. Picture-word cards for production practice are developed next. The child colors (or draws) at least one picture from the four or five carefully selected production-practice words (controlled for phonetic environment) on large (5"x 8") index cards. The child says each word prior to its being selected as a target word for the session so that it can be evaluated for possible assimilation effects and also for the level of difficulty of a particular word for that child. The word is written on the card, which allows adults to identify the picture and also serves to increase the child's awareness of grapheme-phoneme relationships, ultimately contributing to the enhancement of early literacy skills. Some beginning writers like to print the words themselves.

4. The child participates in **experiential-play** production-practice activities. In order to "take a turn," the child names the picture incorporating the target pattern for the session. Models and/or tactile cues are provided as needed (particularly during the first couple of cycles) so that the child achieves 100% success on the target pattern for these

carefully selected production-practice words. Opportunities also are provided for some conversation during each session in order to observe when phonological patterns are beginning to emerge in spontaneous utterances.

5. Next, **stimulability** within the designated target pattern is evaluated to determine the next session's target phoneme. For example, if /s/ clusters are to be targeted the following week, the child is asked to say words such as *spot, stop, smoke, snow, sky,* and/or *boats, tops, books.* Tactile cues and amplification are incorporated if needed. The most stimulable /s/ cluster is selected to be the target for the following session, the next most stimulable /s/ cluster is targeted the next session, and so on.

6. **Phonological awareness** activities (e.g., rhyming, syllable segmentation) are incorporated for a few minutes during each session to help children who may be "at risk" for developing literacy skills because of underlying **phonological representation** deficiencies (see Mody, 2003; Stackhouse, 1997). Sometimes a folder with a four-line rhyme (e.g., "Jack and Jill") that has been read aloud by the clinician is given to the child to take home. A brief phonological awareness assessment tool is often administered to help identify any particular areas that need facilitation. The amount of intervention session time devoted to enhancing phonological awareness skills is often increased during the final cycles.

7. At the end of the session, the listening activity is repeated (again incorporating slight amplification). The same listening list of words that was used at the beginning of the session is read to the child again.

What Is the "Home" Program?

The caregiver (or a paraprofessional) is asked to participate in a 2-minutes-per-day home (or school) program. Each day, the week's listening list is read to the child, and the child names picture cards containing the week's production-practice words. In addition, the caregiver is asked to read the rhyme to the child each night (pausing to allow the child to "fill in" rhyme words) to facilitate the development of onset and rime awareness.

How Are Production-Practice Words Selected?

Words (rather than nonsense syllables) are used for production practice. Monosyllabic words with facilitative phonetic environments (e.g., Buteau & Hodson, 1989; Kent, 1982) are selected during the first few cycles so that clients can experience immediate success.

Words that contain phonemes produced at the same place of articulation as the substitute phoneme must be avoided during early cycles. For example, target words such as *cat, can, kiss, kite,* and *goat* are inappropriate for children who substitute alveolars for velars (i.e., fronting). Likewise, *lamb, lamp, leaf, lip, rope, robe, roof, robot,* and *rabbit* (i.e., words containing labial consonants and/or round vowels) are not used for production-practice words during early cycles for children who substitute the labial glide /w/ for liquids (i.e., gliding). Care must be taken to reduce opportunities for assimilation effects, particularly during the first couple of cycles.

Words for which actual objects (e.g., *boats* and *hats* for word-final /ts/) can be used for elicitation are desirable, especially for preschool children. In addition, action words (e.g., *spin, eats)* are often used to add another dimension. It is desirable, of course, that production-practice words be appropriate for each child's vocabulary level.

What Are Typical Production-Practice Activities?

Experiential-play activities (e.g., fishing, bowling) provide motivation for young children. Refer to Appendix C for an array of activity ideas. It is especially beneficial to incorporate pragmatically appropriate activities. For example, a camera can be incorporated for the production-practice word *smile.* Moreover, it is desirable to have some production-practice activities occur outside the intervention room. In general, student clinicians in our phonology clinic average one activity for every 10 minutes. (The same activities can be repeated week after week.) Clinicians are advised to change to the next activity within a session before the child loses interest, even if that client wants to continue certain favorite activities.

The use of **minimal pair** words (e.g., Fairbanks, 1960) for production practice is excellent for children who have sufficient skills to experience success (see Tyler, Edwards, & Saxman, 1987). The word pairs should contrast the child's own deviation with the target phoneme to help the child understand the semantic differences between the error production and the correct word. Explanations of minimal pair differences can be provided even if the child is not yet at a readiness level for productions of the contrasting words. During the final cycles, the use of minimal pairs can be extremely effective in helping children recognize the semantic differences between the error and the target productions.

Confrontation activities may be appropriate in some instances, especially if perseveration is occurring on specific words. Dean and Howell (1986) discussed providing situations in which a child learns through "conflict and reflection." They stated that the child must have an opportunity for discussion with the adult about the "nature of the problem" and that "graded feedback which extends understanding without discouraging" must be provided. One 6-year-old client persisted in saying [wɛs] for *yes* even after she produced /j/ consistently in other words (Hodson, Nonomura, & Zappia, 1989). It was explained to her that if she said "*Wes*" when asked if she wanted an animal cracker during her break, she would not receive her usual treat. She still said [wɛs] in response to the question that day and then did not receive the treat. From then on, she very carefully answered *yes* to such questions. Dean and Howell stressed that the "task must motivate the child." Confrontation activities should be used only for those clients who can readily produce the target and who demonstrate metalinguistic awareness of the phonological aspects involved.

For school-age clients who can read, a short period of oral reading that focuses on the session's target pattern can be incorporated during each session. The material for this activity must be at a reading level that is lower than the current level of the child so that attention and effort can be directed toward the phonological pattern being targeted rather than on reading decoding.

Clinicians should endeavor to select optimal targets and to provide sufficient cues so that clients can experience 100% success on the session's target pattern for the carefully selected production-practice words. At the beginning of sessions, models and some tactile cues typically are provided to assist the child. Cues and assists are faded as the session progresses and as the child gains facility producing the target pattern.

The process of "counting and charting errors," which has been found to be counterproductive, is not advocated for this phonological remediation approach. It has been observed that "taking data" throughout each session not only interferes with naturalistic interactions between clinician and client, but also allows the child to continue making error productions, which provides practice and reinforcement for the inaccurate kinesthetic image and may lead to "fuzzy" phonological representations (see Stackhouse, 1997). Accountability/outcome measures are provided at the end of each cycle by phonological assessment scores (Hodson, 2004a).

Why and How Are Phonological Awareness Activities Incorporated?

Results of a number of recent studies indicate that children with disordered expressive phonological systems experience greater difficulty than most of their peers with typical phonological development on phonological awareness tasks (Bird, Bishop, & Freeman 1995; Clarke-Klein & Hodson, 1995; Gillon, 2000a, 2004; Stackhouse, 1997; Webster & Plante, 1992). Considerable evidence now exists indicating that children with poor phonological awareness skills experience greater difficulty acquiring literacy (Blachman, 1984; Bradley & Bryant, 1983; Lundberg, Olofsson, & Wall, 1980; Vellutino & Scanlon, 1987). Therefore, developing phonological awareness not only has an impact on a child's phonological productions, but also on his or her literacy skills.

Several projects were implemented in our university clinic in the 1990s to enhance phonological awareness skills of:

- A group of three preschool clients (Domnick, Coffman, Hodson, & Wynne, 1998)
- A group of five kindergarten clients (Hodson, Buckendorf, Conrad, & Swanson, 1994)
- A group of four first-grade clients (Johnson, 1996)
- A group of four second-graders who were former clients (Shields, 1997)

Prior to intervention, phonological awareness and emergent literacy scores of the children lagged behind scores of their peers with typical phonological development. Following intervention, all of the participants evidenced considerable gains, with post-intervention scores approximating scores of their peers.

Some phonological awareness tasks (e.g., rhyming, syllable segmentation, blending, and manipulation) are now being incorporated regularly into clinical sessions. For example, because highly unintelligible clients typically evidence poorer rhyming skills than their peers with typical phonological development (Smith, Kneil, Hodson, Bernstorf, & Gladhart, 1994) and because results of several studies indicate that rhyming is an important early phonological awareness skill (Anthony & Lonigan, 2004; Bryant, MacLean, Bradley, & Crossland, 1990), rhyming activities are incorporated into early phonological remediation sessions. Typically, a folder containing a four-line rhyme (e.g., "Humpty Dumpty") is sent home for parents to read nightly for a period of 2 or 3 weeks per rhyme. The parents are asked to pause and let the child "fill in" the appropriate rhyme word. Syllable segmentation is facilitated by having the child hop for each syllable in a word.

Components from *Animated Literacy* (Stone, 1995), a comprehensive, multisensory early literacy program that blends whole language and phonological awareness are sometimes incorporated (Hodson, 1994b). Phonemic awareness tasks (e.g., phoneme blending and manipulation) are now included in sessions for kindergarten and primary-grade children. (See Chapter 8 for further information about phonological awareness activities.)

When and Why Is Focused Auditory Stimulation Used?

Some children need to begin intervention one step below production practice. For clients who lack stimulability or who are unwilling to participate in production-practice activities (e.g., 2-year-olds), it is recommended that focused auditory stimulation be provided for the first cycle of intervention. Deficient patterns are facilitated in succession by presenting a new phoneme (within a target pattern) during each session.

The child participates in activities and listens, but productions are not expected during this cycle. The clinician talks about selected objects (e.g., *cup, top* for final consonant stimulation) and incorporates activities (e.g., *jump, up)* related to the week's target pattern. All of the deficient patterns (including liquids) are presented auditorily for a cycle. Production-practice activities are incorporated during ensuing cycles (i.e., after the child demonstrates sufficient readiness and willingness).

Theoretical & Conceptual Considerations

What Theoretical/Conceptual Aspects Influenced the Cycles Phonological Remediation Approach?

The Cycles Approach is based on **developmental phonology theories** (e.g., Browman & Goldstein, 1986; Macken & Ferguson, 1983; Stampe, 1972), **cognitive psychology** principles (e.g., Hunt, 1961; Vygotsky, 1962), phonological acquisition research (e.g., Dyson & Paden, 1983; Grunwell, 1987; Ingram, 1976; Porter & Hodson, 2001; Preisser et al., 1988; Stoel-Gammon & Dunn, 1985), and also ongoing clinical phonology research. The theory that the Cycles Approach is most closely aligned with is **gestural phonology** (Browman & Goldstein, 1986; Kent, 1997). The term *gesture* refers to a class of articulatory movements. A basic tenet of gestural phonology theory is that phonological representation is based on speech perception, as well as speech production physical constraints. Gestural phonology has implications/applications for phonological awareness and literacy, as well as for phonological production. According to Mody (2003), literacy acquisition appears to be related to the "integration of recurrent gestural patterns into segmental units" (p. 33). She recommended that intervention methods for literacy acquisition combine metaphonological skill enhancement with production tasks.

It also needs to be mentioned that some of the early targets that are selected during beginning cycles (e.g., /s/ clusters before /s/ singletons; liquids) are compatible with "implicational principles" of generative phonology. The rationale for our early targeting of patterns/phonemes that generally are referred to as "later developing" (e.g., /s/ clusters), however, is based on clinical research findings (discussed earlier in the section on selecting targets), rather than on the research of Gierut and her colleagues (Elbert & Gierut, 1986; Gierut, Morrisette, Hughes, & Rowland, 1996) who recommend, based on their single-subject design studies, that "least phonological knowledge" phonemes should be targeted first. (Note: Results of a randomized controlled experimental study by Rvachew and Nowak [2001] did not support the contention that least phonological knowledge phonemes should be targeted first).

What Underlying Concepts Guide the Cycles Approach?

Seven underlying concepts that serve as the basis for Cycles Approach intervention decisions are listed in Table 6.4. One of the most important concepts is that

Table 6.4

Underlying Concepts of the Cycles Approach

1. Phonological acquisition is a gradual process.
2. Children with "normal" hearing typically acquire the adult sound system primarily by listening.
3. Children associate kinesthetic and auditory sensations as they acquire new patterns, enabling later self-monitoring.
4. Phonetic environment can facilitate (or inhibit) correct sound production.
5. Children are actively involved in their phonological acquisition.
6. Children tend to generalize new speech production skills to other targets.
7. An optimal "match" facilitates a child's learning.

Source: Hodson (1997)

phonological acquisition is gradual (Ingram, 1976). Children with typical development do not learn "one phoneme at a time" (e.g., /f/) to a criterion (e.g., 90%). The Cycles Approach more closely approximates the way in which normal phonological development occurs (Ingram, 1986). Individual phonemes are used to facilitate the development of intelligible speech patterns.

Another critical underlying concept pertains to speech perception. Children with "normal" hearing typically acquire the speech patterns of their linguistic community primarily by listening. Most parents do not teach their children where to place their tongues to make speech sounds. We have found that it is important to incorporate auditory stimulation (see Van Riper, 1939) with slight amplification (Elliott, Longinetti, Clifton, & Meyer, 1981) to help children become aware of the acoustic characteristics of sounds they are not yet producing. Theoretical support for auditory stimulation has been provided by Ingram's (1986) cross-linguistic research. His findings indicate that children first acquire those phonemes to which they have most frequent exposure. Thus, increasing a child's exposure to a phoneme/pattern is likely to increase the prospect of its being acquired.

Production-practice words with **facilitative phonetic environments** (Buteau & Hodson, 1989; Kent, 1982) must be selected, particularly during the beginning cycles. The purpose of production practice is to help clients develop new accurate **kinesthetic** images (Fairbanks, 1954) and adequate articulatory gestures (Kent, 1997) to match with the new auditory images for the eventual purpose of self-monitoring.

Another important underlying concept pertains to selecting an **optimal match** (Hunt, 1961). The reason for conducting phonological assessment/analysis is to determine at what level the child's phonological system is breaking down so that intervention can be initiated one step above the child's current level of functioning. This allows the child to be optimally challenged and yet experience success.

It has been known for some time that it is not necessary to target every deficient sound, because children do tend to **generalize** (McReynolds & Bennett, 1972). What is critical, however, is to select target phonemes/patterns that will "trigger" the most extensive generalization. For example, targeting /s/ clusters before singleton stridents has far-reaching effects. Most preschool children generalize to other singleton stridents after /s/ clusters begin to emerge in conversation.

The child's interactive participation (mental and physical) is an integral component of this approach. Results from child psychology and brain research studies indicate that children learn best when they are actively involved.

What Published Evidence Is Available Regarding Effectiveness of Targeting and Cycling Phonological Patterns?

Almost and Rosenbaum (1998) conducted a randomized controlled intervention study. Twenty-six children who received a phonological assessment rating of "severe" (based on Hodson, 1986a) were assigned randomly to either an immediate intervention group (4 months of intervention followed by 4 months of no intervention) or to a control/delayed intervention group (no intervention for 4 months followed by 4 months of intervention). Four to six phonological patterns selected as potential targets for each child were presented in a modified cycles (Hodson & Paden, 1991) format. Following the first 4 months of the study, results revealed significantly different phonological scores on three measures (Assessment of Phonological Processes–Revised, Hodson, 1986a; Goldman-Fristoe Test of Articulation, Goldman & Fristoe, 1969; Percentage of Consonants Correct, PCC, Shriberg & Kwiatkowski, 1982), with the immediate intervention group obtaining higher scores. At the end of 8 months, scores of the immediate intervention group continued to be significantly better.

In addition, there have been a number of peer-reviewed published case studies that have provided pre- and post-intervention data, as well as details about the clients and their intervention specifics (Gordon-Brannan, Hodson, & Wynne,

1992; Hodson, 1983, 1994a, 2001; Hodson, Chin, Redmond, & Simpson, 1983; Hodson, Nonomura, & Zappia, 1989; Hodson & Paden, 1983, 1991). Although case studies do not provide efficacy evidence, they do yield a measure of feasibility and also may provide an impetus for large-scale efficacy studies (Fey, 2004).

Additional Considerations

The Cycles Phonological Remediation Approach was designed for children with highly unintelligible speech who have the potential for oral communication. Some children, however, do not have the potential for speech. These children, of course, need an alternative/augmentative communication system, rather than direct speech production intervention.

Furthermore, some children do not need pattern-oriented phonological intervention. Phoneme-oriented programs (see Chapter 5) appear to be adequate for children with mild speech disorders who demonstrate only a few essentially intelligible misarticulations (e.g., lisps, /f/ for /θ/). Another known fact is that virtually all intervention methods help children improve (Ingram, 1983), as does maturation. The amount of time required for children with disordered phonological systems to achieve intelligibility, however, varies considerably from one approach to another. Phoneme-oriented programs have been found to be inordinately time consuming for children with severe/profound expressive phonological impairments, often requiring 4 years (or more) to "master" deficient phonemes one at a time (personal communications).

The primary strength of the Cycles Approach is its efficiency (Hodson, 1982, 1997; Hodson & Paden, 1991). Many preschool children have required less than a year of phonological intervention to become intelligible. Typically, three or four cycles (requiring approximately 30 to 40 hours of a speech-language practitioner's contact time) are required for children with severe expressive phonological impairments to become intelligible. The longest amount of contact time required for clients with extremely disordered phonological systems (who were within normal limits cognitively and neurologically) to become **intelligible** (not perfect) via the Cycles Approach has been 65 hours over a period of approximately 2 years (e.g., Hodson, 1982, 1994a, 1997, 2005). A second strength of the Cycles Approach is its adaptability. This approach has been used effectively with groups (e.g., Montgomery & Bonderman, 1989) and with children who have additional etiological issues, such as repaired cleft palate (e.g., Hodson et al., 1983), and childhood apraxia of speech (e.g., Hodson & Paden, 1983, 1991).

This intervention approach also has been used successfully for children with recurrent otitis media, the most common etiological factor reported in case histories of clients with severe speech disorders (Churchill, Hodson, Jones, & Novak, 1988), as well as for children with mild/moderate (Gordon-Brannan et al., 1992) and severe hearing impairment (Garrett, 1986) and also for a child with a cochlear implant (Hodson, 2001). Phonological intervention procedures for children with severe/profound hearing losses need to incorporate suprasegmental aspects (e.g., phrasing, intonation), as well as the typical phonological pattern targets (e.g., /s/ clusters).

The Cycles Approach also has been adapted for individuals with cognitive delays (e.g., Berman, 2001). Time allotments, however, typically have been doubled for these clients. Each phoneme per pattern is targeted for 2 hours, rather than 1 hour. Furthermore, 3 or more years may be required before comparable intelligibility gains are observed. It is of utmost importance that a systematic pattern approach be used for individuals who lack the cognitive abilities to organize into patterns isolated phonemes that were targeted one-by-one.

Considerably more research is needed to determine how this phonological remediation approach can be adapted for use with children who speak languages other than English (Mann & Hodson, 1994). Phonological assessment/analysis procedures are available for other languages (e.g., Froehlich, Hodson, & Edwards, 2001; Hodson, 1986b), but hypotheses need to be formulated and tested to determine optimal intervention modifications and implementations for specific languages.

Summary

The phonological remediation approach described in this chapter incorporates cycles to facilitate the development of intelligible speech patterns in children with disordered phonological systems. Phonological patterns are targeted in succession by using carefully selected production-practice words to help children with expressive phonological impairments develop appropriate articulatory gestures and accurate underlying phonological representations. Deficient phonological patterns are recycled as many times as needed until the targeted patterns begin to emerge in the child's spontaneous conversational utterances. The ordering of phonological patterns within cycles is based on developmental and clinical phonology research findings and on each individual child's phonological abilities.

CHAPTER 7

Client Example—Phonological Intervention

Barbara Williams Hodson

Evaluation

- What Were the Phonological Assessment Results?
- What Additional Diagnostic Information Was Obtained?
- What Were the Outcomes of the Evaluation?

Intervention

- What Were the Phonological Goals?
- What Patterns and Phonemes Were Targeted during the Four Cycles of Phonological Remediation?
- How Were Phonological Awareness Skills Enhanced?
- What Were the Phonological Assessment Results over Time?
- What Were the Recommendations?

Summary & Additional Considerations

Joey (not his real name) was brought to our University Clinic at the age of 3:5:15 (years:months:days) by his mother because of concerns regarding intelligibility. Birth and medical histories were unremarkable except for chronic upper respiratory infections and recurrent otitis media. Joey's parents were well-educated professionals. His brother was 18 months younger than Joey.

Evaluation

What Were the Phonological Assessment Results?

Scores obtained from the Hodson Assessment of Phonological Patterns–3rd edition (HAPP–3; Hodson, 2004) at age 3:6 are provided in Tables 7.1 and 7.2. At the time of this initial assessment, Joey did not produce any (1) final consonants, (2) consonant clusters/sequences, (3) stridents, (4) velars, or (5) liquids.

He did produce the appropriate number of syllables in HAPP–3 stimulus words, but many of the productions were reduplications (e.g., *jumping* → /toto/). His consonant inventory consisted of /p/, /b/, /t/, /d/, /m/, /n/, /w/, and /j/. Most vowel targets were neutralized to /ɑ/, /ʊ/, /ʌ/, or /o/. The only HAPP–3 stimulus word produced correctly during the initial evaluation was *yoyo.* Many of Joey's spontaneous utterances were lengthy. The only word that could be identified at this time, however, was *Daddy.* His overall percentage of intelligible words was less than 5%. The Total (number of) Occurrences of Major Phonological Deviations (TOMPD) score of 195 placed his phonological performance in the High Profound level of severity. (TOMPD Severity Intervals are: 1–50 = Mild; 51–100 = Moderate; 101–150 = Severe; > 150 = Profound [the top 10 points in each interval are specified as high; the bottom 10 points as low].)

Models, tactile cues, and amplification were incorporated for stimulability testing. At the time of the initial evaluation, Joey was stimulable for word-final consonants /p/ and /t/ and for word-initial consonant clusters /sp/ and /st/. Velars and liquids were not stimulable at the time of this evaluation.

What Additional Diagnostic Information Was Obtained?

Results of other evaluations (formal and informal) during the initial assessment and after intervention began indicated that receptive language and general functioning were within normal limits. His scores for the Test for Auditory Comprehension of Language–3rd edition (TACL–3; Carrow-Woolfolk, 1999) placed his performance in the superior range. Results of an oral mechanism examination indicated that structure and function were generally adequate for speech purposes, but poor tongue motility was observed. In addition, it was noted that his breathing was "unusually noisy." Results of audiological testing led to a recommendation for an evaluation by an otolaryngologist. An adenoidectomy

Table 7.1 Major Phonological Deviations HAPP–3 Preintervention Scores (at Age 3:6)

Phonological Deviation	Occurrence Percentages
Omissions	
Syllables	0
Consonant Clusters/Sequences	118*
Consonant Singletons	
• Prevocalic	0
• Intervocalic	7
• Postvocalic	100
Consonant Category Deficiencies	
Sonorants	
• Liquids	100
• Nasals	76
• Glides	60
Obstruents	
• Stridents	100
• Velars	100
• Other (Anterior Nonstridents/Backing)	33
Total Occurrences of Major Phonological Deviations (TOMPD)	195

* The percentage for Consonant Sequence Omissions exceeds 100% if all consonants of any cluster/sequence are omitted (rather than being reduced with at least one consonant remaining).

From *Enhancing Phonological and Metaphonological Skills of Children with Highly Unintelligible Speech* (p. 28), by B. W. Hodson, 2005, Rockville, MD: American Speech-Language-Hearing Association (ASHA). © 2005 by ASHA. Adapted with permission.

Table 7.2 Major Substitutions and Other Strategies HAPP–3 Preintervention Scores (at Age 3:6)

Phonological Deviation	Number ofOccurrences
Vowel Alterations (Phonemic)	31
Stopping	16
Fronting	12
Gliding	12
Reduplication	10
Labial Assimilation	7

From *Enhancing Phonological and Metaphonological Skills of Children with Highly Unintelligible Speech* (p. 29), by B. W. Hodson, 2005, Rockville, MD: American Speech-Language-Hearing Association (ASHA). © 2005 by ASHA. Adapted with permission.

was performed during the summer (age 3:9), and pressure equalizing tubes were inserted bilaterally.

What Were the Outcomes of the Evaluation?

It was concluded that the prognosis for Joey's development of intelligible speech was favorable. Phonological intervention was recommended. His parents requested services be provided at the University Phonology Clinic. Joey began attending weekly 60-minute sessions during the middle of the spring semester at age 3:6.

Intervention

What Were the Phonological Goals?

Results of Joey's initial HAPP–3 (see Table 7.1) indicated that the phonological deviations above 40% included (1) consonant clusters/sequences, (2) postvocalic singletons, (3) stridents, (4) velars, (5) liquids, (6) nasals, and (7) glides.

A review of his transcribed productions on the HAPP–3 recording form revealed that Joey produced prevocalic nasals /m/ and /n/ and glides /w/ and /j/ adequately; therefore, glides and nasals were not specified as targets for beginning cycles. His initial goal statement was to enhance his phonological system and increase intelligibility by facilitating emergence of the following primary phonological patterns:

- postvocalic singletons
- /s/ clusters (i.e., strident and consonant sequences)
- velars
- liquids

(NOTE: See Table 6.1, page 90, for a review of primary target patterns for beginning cycles.)

What Patterns and Phonemes Were Targeted during the Four Cycles of Phonological Remediation?

Cycle One encompassed 7 weekly 60-minute sessions during the second half of the spring semester and 10 sessions during the fall semester. (The University Phonology Clinic was not available during the summer session.) Joey's first Cycle One target pattern was postvocalic singleton consonants, with word-final /p/ and /t/ targeted for 1 hour each. The second target pattern was /s/ clusters. Word-initial /sp/ and /st/ and word-final /ts/ and /ps/ were presented for 1 hour each during the spring semester. The last pattern targeted that semester was velars (anterior/posterior contrasts), with word-final /k/ presented for 1 hour. Velars were continued in the fall semester, with word-initial /k/ and /g/ presented for 1 hour each. /s/ clusters were targeted again during the fall semester, with /sn/, /sm/, and /sk/ being introduced, and /sp/ and /st/ being re-presented (i.e., five weekly 1-hour sessions targeting /s/ clusters). The final target pattern for Cycle One at the end of the fall semester was liquids, with /l/, /r/, and /kr/ targeted for 1 hour each.

/s/ clusters and liquids were recycled during the first 9 sessions of Cycle Two. For the first session, /sp/ and /st/ were grouped together, /sm/ and /sn/ for the second session, followed by /sk/ the third session. Liquids were targeted for 4 sessions, with /l/, /r/, /kr/, and /gr/ presented for 1 hour each. /s/ clusters were recycled again for weeks 8 and 9 in the phrase "It's a _____" (e.g., It's a *spoon).* At this time, it was noted that Joey was generalizing productions of final consonants (i.e., word endings), velars, and /s/ clusters into his conversational speech. It was decided that secondary patterns would be presented for the remainder of Cycle Two, including targeting glide clusters and medial and final /s/ plus stop consonant sequences. The targets were /kw/ (e.g., *queen)* for week 10 and /kj/ (e.g., *cube)* for week 11. Medial /st/ (e.g., *toaster)* was targeted week 12 and final /st/ (e.g., *nest)* week 13.

During the 13 Cycle Three sessions (fall semester) and the 9 Cycle Four sessions (spring semester), liquids and consonant clusters/sequences were recycled, including three-consonant clusters (e.g., /str/). In addition, palatal sibilants (e.g., /ʃ/) were added as targets.

How Were Phonological Awareness Skills Enhanced?

Activities to enhance rhyming skills and to practice segmenting and blending at the syllable level were incorporated in the intervention sessions for short periods (see Chapter 8 for examples of activities). In addition, Joey's family played games at home that involved rhyming and syllable-level activities.

What Were the Phonological Assessment Results over Time?

Preintervention (age 3:6), interim (age 4:7), and post-intervention (age 5:7) data (based on HAPP–3) are provided in Table 7.3. Total Occurrences of Major Phonological Deviations (TOMPD) prior to intervention and at the end of each of the four cycles are depicted in Figure 7.1. In addition, Joey's productions of 10 HAPP–3 stimulus words over time are provided in Table 7.4. It is important to notice the changes that he made in his productions as his phonological system improved. In particular, omissions decreased and substitutions became more appropriate at ages 4:2 and 4:7. At age 5:7, the only phonological deviations that occurred in productions of these words were liquid gliding and vowelization and one example of stopping ([b] for /v/ in *television).*

At age 4:7, percentages of occurrence were below 40% for all of the deviations except liquids. (Even though liquids are facilitated for preschoolers in the Cycles Approach, liquid scores typically lag behind other scores.) The TOMPD was now 30, which placed Joey's phonological performance in the Mild range of severity.

Table 7.3 *Preintervention, Interim, and Post-Intervention HAPP–3 Phonological Assessment Results*

Phonological Deviation	Chronological Age		
	3:6	4:7	5:7
Omissions	Percentages of Occurrence		
• Consonant Clusters/Sequences	118%	62%	18%
• Postvocalic Consonant Singletons	100%	0%	0%
Consonant Category Deficiencies			
• Liquids	100%	100%	95%
• Stridents	100%	10%	5%
• Velars	100%	50%	5%
TOMPD	195	65	30
Severity Interval Level	High Profound	Moderate	Mild

From *Enhancing Phonological and Metaphonological Skills of Children with Highly Unintelligible Speech* (p. 34), by B. W. Hodson, 2005, Rockville, MD: American Speech-Language-Hearing Association (ASHA). © 2005 by ASHA. Adapted with permission.

Figure 7.1 *Total Occurrences of Major Phonological Deviations [TOMPD] Ages 3:6 to 5:7*

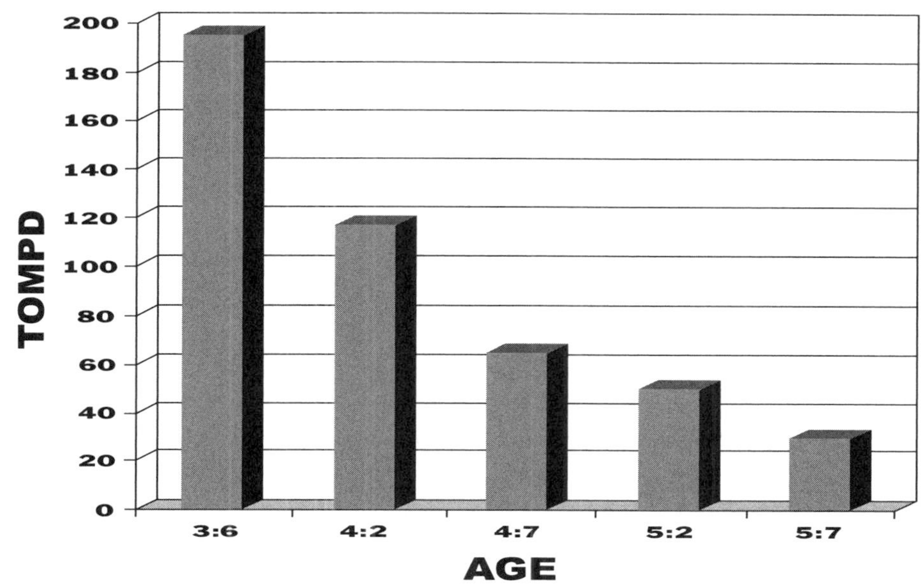

From *Enhancing Phonological and Metaphonological Skills of Children with Highly Unintelligible Speech* (p. 35), by B. W. Hodson, 2005, Rockville, MD: American Speech-Language-Hearing Association (ASHA). © 2005 by ASHA. Adapted with permission.

Table 7.4 *Phonetic Transcriptions of Productions of 10 HAPP–3 Stimulus Words over Time*

Stimulus Word	*Chronological Age*			
	3:6	4:2	4:7	5:7
basket	bɑpə	bæjɪ	bæsɪt	bæskɪt
cowboy hat	tɑtəɑ	taʊbehæt	kaʊbehæt	kaʊbɔɪhæt
glasses	dɑtʊ	dæjɪ	dætɪs	gwæsɪz
hanger	jojə	heŋgʊ	heŋʊ	heŋʊ
ice cubes	ɑpu	aɪtup	aɪtups	aɪskjubz
music box	mowɪbɑ	mudɪbɑk	musɪbɑks	mjuzɪkbɑks
smoke	po	moʊk	smoʊk	smoʊk
soap	po	toʊp	soʊp	soʊp
square	pɛ	pio	sɛə	skwɛʊ
television	jʌjəjojo	tɛjə ɪʤən	tɛwəsɪsən	tɛwəbɪʃən

What Were the Recommendations?

Criteria for dismissal from the University Phonology Clinic for preschoolers require that all of the deviation percentages of occurrence (except liquids) be below 40% and that the TOMPD be below 50. Consequently, recommendations were:

1. Dismissal from the University Phonology Clinic
2. Participation in a 6-week summer program (2 hours twice per week) designed to enhance phonological awareness skills and increase alphabetic principle knowledge to help prepare Joey for kindergarten in the fall
3. Re-evaluation in 6 months

Summary & Additional Considerations

Assessment results before and after four cycles of phonological remediation and phonological targets (patterns and phonemes) for a child whose speech was highly unintelligible at age 3:6 (encompassing 52 contact intervention hours over 25 months) were reported in this chapter. (For additional information and videos on this client, see Hodson, 2005.) Joey was dismissed from the University Phonology Clinic because his speech became essentially intelligible (but not perfect). During the first kindergarten parent conference, his teacher reported that Joey was "exceeding expectations" academically.

It is important to remember that each child's phonological remediation plan must be individualized. A second important consideration is that early intervention is critical for children like Joey to help prepare them for success in school. A third consideration pertains to the importance of enhancing phonological patterns, with phonemes being used as a means to an end (rather than focusing on mastery of each phoneme).

CHAPTER 8

Phonological Awareness—Implications for Children with Expressive Phonological Impairment

Gail T. Gillon

Basic Considerations

- What Is Phonological Awareness?
- How Does Phonological Awareness Develop?
- What Factors Influence Phonological Awareness Development During the Preschool Years?

Phonological Awareness Abilities in Children with Highly Unintelligible Speech

- Why Is It Important to Examine Phonological Awareness During the Preschool Years?
- What Is the Critical Age Hypothesis?

Phonological Awareness Assessment

- What Are the Aims of Assessments Used for Young Children?
- What Assessment Tasks Can Be Used with Young Children?
- What Special Considerations Should Be Given to the Assessment of Young Children with Expressive Phonological Impairment?

Phonological Awareness Intervention

- Is There Evidence That Phonological Awareness Intervention Is Effective?
- What Is the Goal of Phonological Awareness Intervention for Young Children?
- What Approaches Can Be Used to Facilitate Development of Early Phoneme Awareness?
- What Type of Activities Can Facilitate Phoneme Awareness?

Summary

Basic Considerations

Learning to read and spell an alphabetic language requires children to understand that spoken words comprise smaller sound units and that letters on a page can represent these speech sounds. This conscious awareness of the sound structure of words, referred to as **phonological awareness** (or **metaphonological awareness),** is critical for literacy acquisition. Without phonological awareness, children are forced to rely on reading by a whole-word strategy through memorizing the visual image of a printed word to its spoken counterpart. Research has demonstrated that this strategy is inefficient. Children who depend on visual memorization when reading are likely to be the poorest readers, even by the second year of schooling (Stuart, 1995). In contrast, children who have strong phonological awareness skills and letter knowledge are more likely to demonstrate positive outcomes from early literacy instruction (Torgesen, Wagner, & Rashotte, 1994). Measures of young children's phonological awareness are more strongly related to later reading and spelling ability than factors such as socioeconomic status and general language performance (MacDonald & Cornwall, 1995; Share, Jorm, MacLean, & Matthews, 1984). How, then, do children become consciously aware of a word's phonological structure and learn to use phonological information when reading and spelling? Why do children with **expressive phonological impairment** typically struggle to develop this knowledge? This chapter explores the development of early phonological awareness and addresses phonological awareness assessment and intervention issues for children with expressive phonological impairment.

What Is Phonological Awareness?

The term phonological awareness was introduced into the literature in the late 1970s and early 1980s (e.g., Bradley & Bryant, 1983) and may be defined as the awareness of the sound structure of spoken words. Phonological awareness is one aspect of the broader category of metalinguistics and thus is sometimes also referred to as metaphonological awareness. Metalinguistic knowledge refers to a child's ability to reflect upon and discuss aspects of language separate from the meaning of the language. For example, phonological awareness requires a child to reflect upon a word's sound structure as a separate activity from understanding the word's meaning. Mattingly (1972) was among the first to suggest that a relationship exists between children's metalinguistic awareness of language and their development of reading. Researchers have subsequently demonstrated that semantic, syntactic, and morphological awareness also influences reading and spelling development (Bowey, 1986; Carlisle, 1995; Scarborough, 1990).

Phonological awareness may also be seen as a subset of more general phonological processing ability. Wagner and Torgesen (1987) described how the storage and retrieval of phonological information in memory could be viewed as differing constructs of phonological awareness. These researchers used **phonological processing** as an umbrella term that encompasses phonological awareness, but includes other phonological skill areas that are necessary for children to use phonological information in the reading and spelling process.

Phonological awareness reflects knowledge of the phonological structure of a word. Just as a word can be analyzed at the syllable, onset-rime, and phoneme level, so too does the term phonological awareness encompass awareness of syllables, **onsets and rimes,** and **phonemes** within words. For example:

- Phonological awareness at the syllable level is demonstrated when a child identifies syllables within a word (such as clapping out three syllables in the word *butterfly: but - ter - fly).*

- Children demonstrate phonological awareness at the onset-rime level when they show awareness that the onset of a syllable (i.e., the consonant(s) that precede the vowel) can be separated from the rime unit (i.e., the vowel and following consonants). When children recognize that *cat, hat, mat,* and *bat* are rhyming words or when they blend or segment words at the onset-rime level (e.g., *fr* [onset] + *og* [rime] = *frog),* they show an awareness of onset-rime units within words.

- Phonological awareness at the phoneme level (commonly referred to as **phoneme awareness** or **phonemic awareness)** is demonstrated when children identify or recognize individual phonemes in a word, such as identifying a sound within a word (e.g., *sun* ends with /n/), counting the number of phonemes within a word (e.g., *ship* has three sounds: /ʃ/ /ɪ/ /p/), deleting a phoneme from a word (e.g., deleting /k/ from *cup* to make *up),* or blending phonemes together to form a word (e.g., *s-t-o-p* = *stop).*

How Does Phonological Awareness Develop?

A developmental progression from awareness of larger to smaller sound units within words is apparent. Although exceptions to this pattern have been reported in the literature (Duncan & Johnston, 1999), most children demonstrate awareness of syllables and onset-rime units prior to demonstrating awareness of phonemes (Carroll, Snowling, Hulme, & Stevenson, 2003). Wide variability in preschool children's development in phonological awareness is evident. Some children can demonstrate phonological awareness as young as 2 and 3 years of age (Lonigan, Burgess, Anthony, & Barker, 1998). Others are only just beginning to acquire these skills at 4 and 5 years (Dodd & Gillon, 2001). The weight of evidence suggests stability in phonological awareness at the syllable and onset-rime level develops between 4 and 5 years of age. Early awareness of phonemes in words (e.g., awareness of word-initial phonemes) is evident in many 4-year-old children, but successful performance on **complex phoneme awareness tasks** (such as **phoneme segmentation** and **phoneme manipulation)** is usually only present in school-age children (i.e., from 6 years or older). Indeed, reading and spelling instruction play a major role in the development of advanced **phoneme awareness** knowledge (Cataldo & Ellis, 1988).

What Factors Influence Phonological Awareness Development During the Preschool Years?

A range of factors influences the emergence of **phonological awareness** in preschool children. These include (1) vocabulary development, (2) early language experiences, and (3) the child's native language.

Vocabulary Development

Metsala (1999a, 1999b) found positive correlations between the size of the child's receptive vocabulary and performance on phonological awareness tasks at the onset-rime and phoneme level for 4-, 5-, and 6-year-old children. Metsala concluded that phonological awareness emerges from basic language (phonological) development and that developmental models of how children recognize spoken words are relevant to understanding the source of phonological awareness. The importance of vocabulary size, however, may only be related in the early years during the period of rapid vocabulary growth. For example, Elbro, Borstrom, and

Petersen (1998) found that vocabulary size at age 6 years did not predict later phoneme awareness performance for Danish-speaking children.

Children's vocabulary development may influence phonological awareness through a "lexical restructuring" process (Walley, Metsala, & Garlock, 2003). This theory holds that as young children's vocabularies develop rapidly, the phonological information related to a spoken word that is stored in memory **(phonological representation)** is restructured from a whole-word representation to one based on segmental units. This reduces memory capacity demand, as only a limited number of phonemes and information about their articulatory features needs to be stored, rather than trying to store every new word as a whole independent unit. It is only when a child's phonological representation of a word is segmental in nature that a child can consciously access sound segments such as syllables, onset-rime units, or phonemes within the word.

The "quality" of a child's phonological representation stored in memory also influences children's phoneme awareness development (Elbro et al., 1998). That is, a child's underlying representation of a spoken word needs to contain sufficient information about the phoneme segments within the word for a child to successfully reflect on its phonological properties.

Early Language Experiences

The wide variability in preschool children's phonological awareness performance suggests that the type of early language experiences to which a child is exposed influences its development. This suggestion is supported through research demonstrating significant differences in phonological awareness development between children in differing socioeconomic groups (Lonigan et al., 1998). Children between 2 and 5 years of age, from middle-income families were observed to perform better on phonological awareness tasks than children from low-socioeconomic families. Differing rates of development were also evident. Children from mid- to high-income families showed accelerated growth in performance from 3 to 4 years of age, and many could demonstrate successful performance on more advanced phoneme-level tasks at 5 years of age. In contrast, children from low-income families showed less growth in phonological awareness development with increasing age, and the majority failed to score above chance levels on rhyme and phoneme level tasks at age 5 years.

An important early language experience that influences phonological awareness development is children's exposure to **alphabet knowledge** (Burgess & Lonigan, 1998; Johnston, Anderson, & Holligan, 1996; Stahl & Murray, 1994). Learning the names of alphabetic letters and their associated common phonemes helps children understand the sound structure of words. Johnston et al. (1996) argued that letter knowledge may be the trigger for phoneme awareness in preschool children because explicit phoneme awareness ability develops after children have gained at least partial alphabetic knowledge. In support of this view, Castles and Coltheart's (2004) comprehensive review of the literature raised the issue as to whether conscious awareness of a phoneme can ever exist independently of letter knowledge.

Adopting a simple linear model from letter knowledge to phoneme awareness to reading is problematic, however. Letter knowledge instruction alone, for example, does not result in improved word decoding (Adams, 1990), and there is evidence that an initial level of phonological awareness is necessary for a child to be able to use **letter-name knowledge** in word recognition (Tunmer, Herriman, & Nesdale, 1988). Further, phoneme awareness makes a unique contribution to predicting reading even when letter knowledge is taken into consideration (Elbro et al., 1998). Thus, there is general support for an important bidirectional relationship, rather than a one-way relationship, between alphabetic knowledge and phoneme awareness development (Burgess & Lonigan, 1998).

Phonological awareness development in young children may also be influenced through more general stimulation of metalinguistic knowledge. Early language experiences that include directing children's attention to print during shared book reading facilitate children's awareness of the relationship between speech and print. Justice and Ezell (2004) described how **print-referencing activities** (such as an adult pointing to words, commenting on specific words or letters on the page, or asking children specific questions about print during the process of reading a story to a child) help children acquire foundational skills for literacy. Books with large bold print or print embedded in illustrations are useful in promoting such activities. Children's awareness of print concepts; knowledge of what a word, letter, or sound is; and letter-name knowledge may be facilitated through print referencing (Ezell & Justice, 2000; Justice & Ezell, 2000). Thus, the positive relationship between alphabetic knowledge and phoneme awareness may be enhanced through shared book reading experiences and the types of storybooks shared.

Other oral language experiences such as teaching children nursery rhymes facilitate early phonological awareness knowledge. For example, Bryant, Bradley, MacLean, and Crossland (1989) found that the abilities of 3-year-old children to recite nursery rhymes was strongly correlated with rhyme awareness at 4 years of age and phoneme awareness at 5 and 6 years of age.

Native Language

The general developmental trend from awareness of syllables and onset-rime units to awareness of phonemes evident in English is also apparent in other alphabetic languages, such as Italian and Spanish (Cossu, Shankweiler, Liberman, Katz, & Tola, 1988; Denton, Hasbrouck, Weaver, & Riccio, 2000). The language the child is exposed to, however, can influence performance on specific phonological awareness tasks. For example, Cossu et al. (1988) observed that Italian-speaking children developed stronger **syllable awareness** skills at an early age compared to English-speaking children. Young children whose first language is Cantonese or Japanese show inferior phonological awareness performance compared to English-speaking children (Cheung, Chen, Lai, Wong, & Hills, 2001; Mann, 1987), and adequate exposure to an alphabetic script, as opposed to a logographic script, is necessary for individuals to be able to use phonological information in the reading and spelling process (Holm & Dodd, 1996).

Phonological Awareness Abilities in Children with Highly Unintelligible Speech

It is well established that school-age children with moderate or severe expressive phonological impairment perform poorly on phonological awareness tasks (Bird, Bishop, & Freeman, 1995; Webster & Plante, 1992). This difficulty may persist well into adolescence (Snowling, Bishop, & Stothard, 2000). The presence of phonological awareness deficits in children with expressive phonological impairment is independent of whether these children have additional receptive and expressive language impairment (Bird et al., 1995; Leitao, Hogben, & Fletcher, 1997), although children who have both speech and language impairments are likely to exhibit weaker phonological awareness performance and have poorer long-term literacy outcomes compared with children who have only expressive phonological impairment (Lewis, Freebairn, & Taylor, 2000; Snowling et al., 2000).

Why Is It Important to Examine Phonological Awareness During the Preschool Years?

Recent investigations have confirmed that differences in phonological awareness development between children with and without speech impairment are evident well before these children commence formal literacy instruction. Thus, their phonological awareness difficulties are not simply a consequence of poor reading. For example, the performance of 4-year-old children with moderate or severe speech impairment was found to be significantly inferior to children with typical speech development on rhyme matching, initial onset matching, and phoneme perception tasks (Rvachew, Ohberg, Grawburg, & Heyding, 2003). The group difference was evident despite the group's being carefully matched for within-average-range performance on a measure of receptive vocabulary. The children with speech impairment did, however, exhibit the same developmental pattern of performance as the children without speech impairment. Rhyme matching proved an easier task than initial onset matching for both groups, and the onset segmentation task was equally challenging for both groups.

Persistent delayed development in the ability to detect rhyme oddity and initial phoneme oddity prior to literacy instruction (i.e., development between the ages of 3 and 6 years) for children with expressive phonological impairment has also been reported (Webster & Plante, 1995). Interestingly, Webster and Plante observed a relationship between children's speech production skills and their success on the phonological awareness tasks. As children's speech error patterns resolved over time from excessive or moderate use of error patterns to milder categories of speech error patterns, the percentage of children who gained a score of 70% or higher on the phonological awareness tasks more than doubled. Their findings suggest that improvement in speech production might be a catalyst for accelerating phonological awareness development. All of the children with expressive phonological impairment in the study were, however, receiving intervention, and detail as to whether the intervention directly facilitated phonological awareness development was not reported.

Subsequent research has indicated that phonological awareness at the syllable and onset-rime level may develop in children with expressive phonological impairment as a consequence of intervention aimed at improving speech intelligibility or through general preschool or classroom instruction, but development at the phoneme awareness level is not as responsive to more general speech and language stimulation. For example, Gillon (2000a, 2002) found that 6-year-old children with expressive phonological impairment required specific **phonological awareness intervention** focused predominantly at the phoneme level (e.g., **phoneme identity, phoneme segmentation, phoneme manipulation,** and **phoneme blending** activities) in order to achieve accelerated gains in phoneme awareness, reading, and spelling performance. Improvement in speech production alone did not necessarily result in significant improvement in phoneme awareness and literacy performance.

Carroll and Snowling (2004) also highlighted the need to consider phonological development in children with expressive phonological impairment beyond the level of speech intelligibility. Investigating the phonological awareness skills of 4- to 6-year-old children, the researchers found similar patterns of poor performance on phonological awareness tasks for children with expressive phonological impairment and children with no overt speech production difficulties, but who had a genetic disposition for dyslexia (i.e., a parent or sibling diagnosed with dyslexia). Both groups showed delayed development in phonological awareness at the onset-rime and phoneme level compared to children without risk factors. Carroll and Snowling concluded that young children with speech impairment and children with a genetic disposition for dyslexia may have a common risk factor in that their underlying phonological representations of words are poorly specified.

A poorly specified representation of a word's phonological structure that a child stores in memory, or difficulty in consciously accessing and retrieving phonological information from a word's representation, restricts the child's ability to understand the relationship between the phonological and orthographic form of word. This, in turn, results in a breakdown in word **decoding** or encoding when reading and spelling. Such difficulties are not necessarily linked to the severity of the child's conversational speech intelligibility because children without speech difficulties and children with mild speech errors (see Cowan & Moran, 1997) can present with the same types of underlying phonological difficulty.

Difficulty in representing, storing, and/or retrieving phonological information may also explain observed bilingual phonological awareness deficits. Martin, Colesby, and Jhamat (1997) discussed how children who have expressive phonological impairment and are learning English as a second language may demonstrate phonological awareness difficulties in both their native and second language. These difficulties may be present despite speech-language intervention that has proven successful in largely resolving their speech disorder, such as the case study of a 7-year-old child reported in Martin et al. (1997). Thus, from a clinical perspective, it is critical that assessment and intervention for children with unintelligible speech not only address speech intelligibility, but also consider other aspects of the child's phonological system, such as his or her phonological awareness development.

What Is the Critical Age Hypothesis?

The importance of examining phonological awareness development in young children with expressive phonological impairment is consistent with the modified "critical age hypothesis" developed in relation to predicting which children with expressive phonological impairment are most at risk for persistent reading and spelling difficulties (Nathan, Stackhouse, Goulandris, & Snowling, 2004). Initially, Bishop and Adams (1990) proposed that if children's speech and language difficulties resolve by the early school years, then they are likely to have positive literacy outcomes. They referred to this prediction as the critical age hypothesis to address the variability observed in reading development for preschool children who presented with isolated speech impairments. Longitudinal and experimental research evidence, however, now indicates that, in addition to resolving children's speech impairment, the level of children's phonological awareness is a critical factor in determining literacy outcomes (Larrivee & Catts, 1999; Nathan et al., 2004). Nathan et al. therefore proposed a modified critical age hypothesis in that literacy outcome may be more positive for preschool children with speech impairment if their speech impairment resolves early and they acquire adequate phoneme awareness knowledge.

Phonological Awareness Assessment

The accurate assessment of phonological awareness in children with unintelligible speech should form a vital component in comprehensive assessment procedures. The assessment of phonological awareness helps profile these children's speech and language development.

What Are the Aims of Assessments Used for Young Children?

Basically, phonological awareness assessment for preschool children with expressive phonological impairment have two purposes. The assessment serves to:

1. Observe the child's current level of phonological awareness performance in order to establish baseline data from which the effectiveness of specific interventions can be measured

2. Monitor whether the child is gaining phonological awareness skills during the preschool years in a manner similar to children with typical development

What Assessment Tasks Can Be Used with Young Children?

A variety of formal and informal assessment tools are available to measure children's phonological awareness development in the preschool and early school years. Some examples are included in Appendix E. Standardized assessment tools that measure a broad range of phonological awareness skills (e.g., Preschool and Primary Inventory of Phonological Awareness, by Dodd, Crosbie, MacIntosh, Teitzel, & Ozanne, 2000) are useful to establish current level of performance and to monitor a child's development when administered periodically during the preschool years, in comparison to a normative database. Informal assessment measures (e.g., the phoneme oddity task developed by Bradley and Bryant, 1983, *"Which word starts with a different sound: hill, pigs, pin?")* and dynamic assessment methods (e.g., *DIBELS*, by Good and Kaminski, 2002, see Appendix E) may be useful in evaluating the effectiveness of specific interventions or monitoring development at more regular intervals than recommended for standardized testing procedures. Assessment measures employed to evaluate intervention effectiveness need to be sufficiently sensitive to identify any change in the skills targeted in intervention; to measure transfer of newly acquired skills to untrained tasks; and, when the child reaches school age, to measure skill transfer to the ability to use phonological information in the reading and spelling process.

What Special Considerations Should Be Given to the Assessment of Young Children with Expressive Phonological Impairment?

In assessing the phonological awareness development of young children with expressive phonological impairment, careful consideration should be given to the type of tasks used and the testing environment. For example:

- Selecting tasks that require nonverbal responses is important for children with unintelligible speech (e.g., *"Point to the picture that starts with* /m/: *mat, dog, book;"* see Gillon, 2000c).
- Ensuring optimal listening conditions in the phonological awareness testing environment is important for all children, but particularly critical for young children with expressive phonological impairment who may have associated hearing problems.
- The use of attractive visual picture cues to supplement an auditory stimulus will help capture young children's attention.
- Ensuring working memory capacity is not overloaded for children who are known to have limited phonological short-term memory is another important consideration. The use of target words with a maximum of three or four phonemes is recommended for these children (Cupples & Iacono, 2000).

The data from phonological awareness assessment need to be considered along with data from comprehensive analyses of the children's speech and language performance. Analyzing data from speech production tasks that include a variety of multisyllabic words and assessment of nonword repetition ability, as suggested by Larivee and Catts (1999); examining the variability in children's speech production errors and the type of speech error patterns, as suggested by Dodd (1995), and Leitao and Fletcher (2004); and examining data related to the children's receptive and expressive language performance alongside data pertaining to the child's phonological awareness abilities will help determine which young children with expressive phonological impairment are most at risk for **literacy difficulties. Preventative intervention** that specifically aims to enhance the phonological awareness development of these children in their preschool and early school years may assist in the prevention of persistent literacy difficulties that these children may otherwise encounter.

Phonological Awareness Intervention

Is There Evidence That Phonological Awareness Intervention Is Effective?

Improving literacy performance for children who struggle to read and write is a goal strongly supported by all literate societies. Research that claims significant benefits from phonological awareness intervention toward enhancing children's literacy development has therefore received intensive scrutiny. The most comprehensive meta-analysis of phonological awareness intervention involved analysis of 52 controlled intervention studies (Ehri et al., 2001). This meta-analysis confirmed that improving children's awareness of the sound structure of words significantly enhances children's word recognition, reading comprehension, and spelling development.

The majority of intervention studies in phonological awareness have examined the benefits of this intervention for general populations of children in regular classrooms or preschools. The last decade, though, has seen the development of research indicating that children at risk can also benefit from phonological awareness instruction. For example, young children at risk from low socioeconomic backgrounds (Blachman, Ball, Black, & Tangel, 1994); children starting school with poor **phonological processing** skills (Castle, Riach, & Nicholson, 1994; Torgesen et al., 1999); and children with spoken language impairment (Gillon, 2000a, 2002) have all demonstrated positive reading and/or spelling outcomes in response to phonological awareness instruction. In a longitudinal study, Gillon (2005) demonstrated that stimulating early phoneme awareness and letter knowledge in children with expressive phonological impairment when they are 3 and 4 years of age, led to a major advantage for the development of these children's word recognition and spelling skills in their early school years.

What Is the Goal of Phonological Awareness Intervention for Young Children?

The aim of phonological awareness intervention for preschool children (i.e., 3- to 5-year-old children) with expressive phonological impairment is to facilitate these children's development to ensure they approach literacy instruction with the foundation skills that will allow them to use phonological information in the reading and spelling process. The focus of the intervention should be on facilitation and not aimed at resolving a deficit or teaching skill mastery of complex phoneme awareness tasks. The wide variability in typical phonological awareness development in this young age group and the known impact of reading and spelling instruction on enhancing more advanced phoneme awareness would make the latter inappropriate.

What Approaches Can Be Used to Facilitate Development of Early Phoneme Awareness?

Differing approaches to facilitating young children's phonological awareness development during the preschool years may be taken. One approach is to ensure that the factors that influence phonological awareness development (as discussed earlier in this chapter) are enhanced. Intervention strategies based on this approach may include:

- Expanding the children's receptive vocabulary knowledge at 3 or 4 years of age if vocabulary development is delayed
- Teaching children nursery rhymes and focusing their attention on the sound properties and rhythms of spoken language
- Facilitating children's exposure to alphabetic knowledge through alphabet books and songs or through print-referencing techniques that draw children's attention to letters on a storybook page
- Facilitating children's general metacognitive development through activities that encourage children to reflect on words and language (e.g., noticing word length in spoken and written form; identifying the rhyming words in a story or poem)

These types of activities can be implemented within early education or home contexts. The speech-language pathologist needs to collaborate with parents, caregivers, and early education teachers to encourage the participation of children with poor speech intelligibility in tasks that enhance knowledge known to influence phonological awareness development.

A second approach to facilitating phonological awareness development in children with expressive phonological impairment is to implement specific teaching activities during these children's intervention to improve their speech intelligibility. Based on research evidence (e.g., Burgess & Lonigan, 1998; Ehri et al., 2001), such an approach should work toward stimulating skills at the phoneme level (i.e., the approach should not focus only on syllable and rhyme knowledge) and should incorporate activities to facilitate letter knowledge. The phoneme awareness and letter knowledge activities may relate directly to the children's speech production goals or may introduce independent phoneme targets that can be interspersed between activities to improve speech intelligibility. The child's speech-language pathologist should implement this approach (with support from the child's caregivers or early education teachers) in a manner that carefully adjusts task difficulty and stimulus items as appropriate to the child's abilities.

What Type of Activities Can Facilitate Phoneme Awareness?

A variety of phoneme awareness and letter knowledge activities can be incorporated into interventions for young children with unintelligible speech. An example of a three-step model to facilitate awareness of the link between speech and print and knowledge that words comprise individual phonemes is provided. The /s/ phoneme is used as a teaching example.

Step 1

Introduce the connection between a target phoneme and its common graphemes **(phoneme-grapheme relationship).** A child is shown a large poster-size letter *s* and instructed that the name of the letter is *s* and the sound it makes is /s/. If appropriate to the child's speech production abilities or teaching goals, the child should be encouraged to articulate /s/ in isolation. For example, *"Throw the bean bag onto the letter* s (a visually distinct letter such as *m* may be used as a distractor item). *Each time the bean bag lands on the letter* s, *let's make /s/ together."*

Step 2

Encourage awareness of the phoneme in spoken words. Introduce activities that encourage awareness of /s/ in word-initial position. For example, using prompting techniques, assist the child to find toys or pictures that start with /s/ from an array of carefully chosen words that have wide initial sound contrasts and (where possible) have phonetically regular spellings like *sun, ball,* and *mat.* Once the target /s/ words have been found, the child is encouraged to model or approximate the correct articulation of the words as appropriate to speech production goals.

Step 3

Facilitate awareness of the relationship between phonemes and graphemes in a word context. Once the child has selected the picture or toy that starts with /s/ (as described in Step 2), write the word in large, plain print on a piece of cardboard and bring the child's attention to the initial letter and sound in the word. Encourage the child to articulate the word again through "reading" the written word. For example:

"This word says "sun." See the letter s *at the beginning of the word? Hear* /s/ *at the start of the word? Let's read the word together: sun. Now, you read the word* sun *to Teddy* (or Mom/Dad) *and place the word* sun *by the picture of the sun."*

Words used in this type of three-step model may include words identified for the child's speech production practice, such as the five target words suggested in the Cycles Phonological Remediation Approach (see Chapter 6). The following are examples of other phoneme awareness activities that may be included in Step 2 of this approach.

Initial Phoneme Identity

Example 1:

"Here is a car. Car *starts with* /k/. *Let's drive the car to another toy that starts with* /k/." (The child has a choice of a cow, a bus, a fish.) Prompt the child as necessary to develop awareness that *car* and *cow* both start with /k/.

Example 2:

"Listen to these words that start with /m/: man, milk, mat, moon. (Encourage the child to listen and watch your articulation of the words.) *What sound does* mail *start with?* (Prompt as necessary to help the child identify the /m/ sound). *Yes* mail *starts with /m/. Let's see what toys that start with /m/ are hiding in the mailbag."* (The child pulls out various parcels from the mailbag. Inside each parcel, the child will find two toys, such as a mouse and a dog. Help the child identify which one of the two toys starts with /m/.)

Final Phoneme Identity

Example 1:

"Here is a yacht. Listen to the /t/ sound at the end of yacht. *Let's sail the yacht to another word that ends with a /t/ sound."* (The child has a choice of a *ship* or a *boat.* Articulate the words *ship* and *boat,* and encourage the child to watch his or her mouth to observe visual cues for the final /t/ sound.)

Example 2:

"Listen to these words that end with /p/: tap, cup, hop loop. (Encourage the child to listen and watch your articulation.) *Let's make this rabbit hop to toys that end with a /p/ sound."* (At each turn, the child has a choice of two objects whose names have wide final phoneme contrasts, such as a *cup* and a *bus.*)

A variety of commercial materials are available to help facilitate young children's conscious awareness that words comprise individual speech sounds (see Appendix F and also see Gillon, 2004). It is important to keep the young child actively engaged in the activity and to select materials or toys that will capture a young child's attention. Integrating phoneme awareness activities with speech production goals will maximize intervention efficiency. The intervention should result in:

- Improved speech intelligibility
- Enhanced phonological awareness skills
- Increased letter knowledge

All of these factors are important for successful reading and spelling experiences when the child begins school.

Young children with expressive phonological impairment should be carefully monitored following school entry and during the early school years. Periods of structured and more intensive phonological awareness intervention may be necessary if the child appears to struggle to use phonological information in the reading and spelling process. Structured programs for at-risk, school-age children should focus predominantly on developing skills at the phoneme level (e.g., activities to develop phoneme identity, phoneme matching, phoneme segmentation, phoneme blending, or phoneme manipulation skills) and should make explicit for the child the link between the phonological and orthographic form of a word. In recent years, there has been a rapid growth in the publication of materials and programs suitable to develop kindergarten and school-age children's phonological awareness abilities. Some programs are designed for classroom-based work, whereas others are suitable for small-group or individualized intervention. Appendix F provides examples of intervention programs and resources. Ensuring that children with expressive phonological impairment have strong phoneme awareness and letter knowledge during their first year at school will assist them in decoding printed words, recognizing printed words, and using phonological cues in spelling words. This, in turn, will facilitate reading fluency and reading comprehension (Stanovich, 1985). Thus, the positive interactions between advancing spoken and written language development evident in children with typical speech and language skills will also be afforded to children with expressive phonological impairment.

Summary

Phonological awareness is critical for successful early reading and spelling development. Conscious awareness that words comprise smaller sound units (syllables, onset-rimes, and phonemes) assists children in printed word recognition and spelling processes. Most children begin to exhibit sensitivity to a word's sound structure during their preschool years, with a range of factors (such as vocabulary development and early language experiences) contributing to the development of this phonological awareness. Children with expressive phonological impairment frequently show delayed development in phonological awareness and experience particular difficulty on phoneme-level tasks. Results of research indicate that such difficulty will restrict these children's early reading and spelling development and highlight the importance of addressing broader aspects of the child's phonological system in assessment and intervention practices. In addition to improving speech intelligibility, early intervention that facilitates phoneme awareness and letter knowledge may help children with expressive phonological impairment experience reading and writing success.

PART IV

Theoretical Considerations, Major Issues & Research Needs

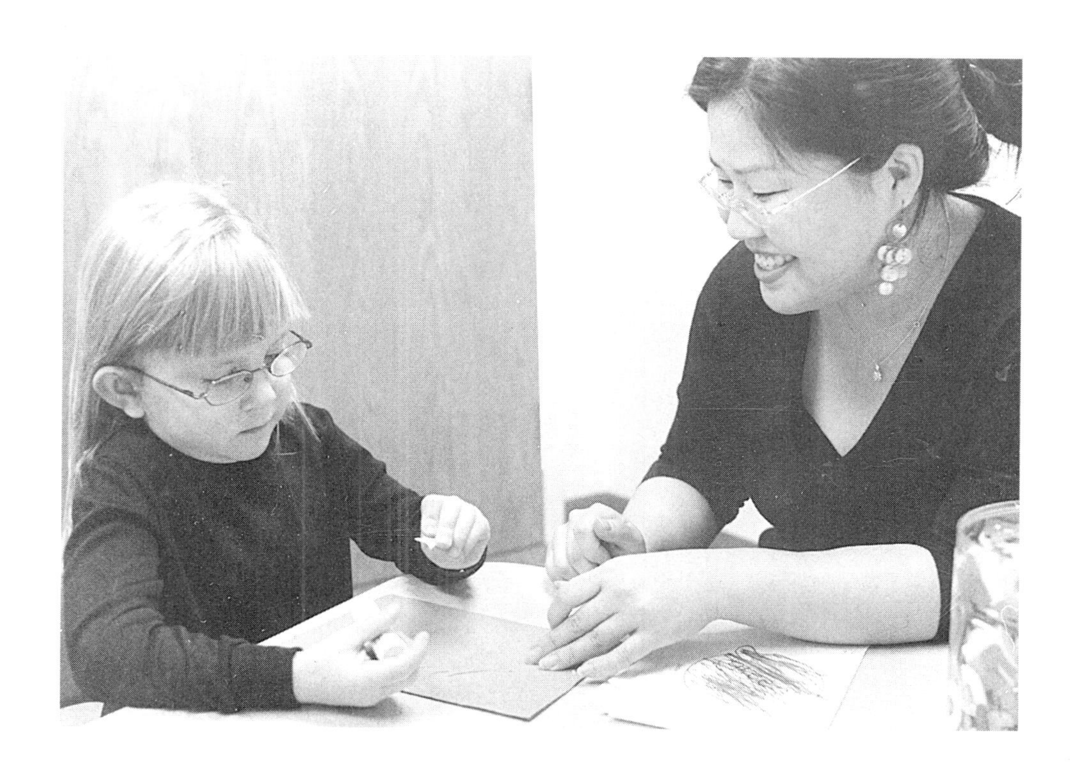

CHAPTER 9

Phonological Theories

Mary Louise Edwards

Descriptive Linguistics

- Characteristics of Descriptive Linguistics
- Clinical Applications of Descriptive Linguistics

Behaviorist Theories

- Autism Theory
- Ease of Perception Theory
- Clinical Applications

Universal Order Theory

- Roman Jakobson
- The Principle of Maximal Contrast
- Implicational Universals
- The Discontinuity View
- Some Strengths and Weaknesses of the Universal Order Theory

Distinctive Feature Theory

- Some Characteristics of Distinctive Feature Theory
- Uses of Distinctive Features
- Markedness
- Clinical Applications of Distinctive Features

Generative Phonology

- Phonological Rules and Applications
- Writing Phonological Rules
- Clinical Applications of Phonological Rules
- Underlying Representations
- Productive Phonological Knowledge
- Clinical Applications of Productive Phonological Knowledge

Natural Phonology

- Natural Phonological Processes
- Stampe's View of Children's Underlying Representations
- Innate Phonological System Revisions
- Clinical Applications of Natural Phonology

Prosodic Theory

- Characteristics of Prosodic Theory
- Clinical Applications of Prosodic Theory

Interactionist-Discovery Theory

- A Discovery-Oriented Approach
- Children Limiting Their Output
- Clinical Applications of Interactionist-Discovery Theory

Nonlinear Theories

- Characteristics of Nonlinear Theories
- Metrical Phonology
- Clinical Applications of Metrical Phonology
- Feature Geometry
- Segments Representation in Feature Geometry
- Clinical Applications of Feature Geometry

Optimality Theory

- Characteristics of Optimality Theory
- Constraints and Ranking
- Constraint Table
- Relationships of Phonological Processes and Constraints
- Clinical Applications of Optimality Theory

Gestural Phonology

- Characteristics of Gestural Phonology
- Gestural Score
- Relationships of Gestures and Phonological Processes
- Clinical Applications of Gestural Phonology

Summary

As part of its linguistic system or "grammar," each language has a **phonological system** consisting of the sounds that are used in that language, along with various types of rules showing how those sounds function and pattern. For example, **phonotactic** rules specify where sounds can occur and how they can be combined. These rules differ from language to language. (Would "srtiksn" be an acceptable word in English?)

Numerous theories have been proposed for how sound systems are organized. Some of these have focused almost entirely on adult languages, whereas others have focused only on children's acquisition of the sound system. A few have attempted to account for both adult phonological systems and phonological acquisition in children. Although each theory accounts for certain phenomena, no single theory accounts for everything, and there has never been one theory on which all experts agree.

This chapter provides an overview of several phonological theories proposed in the 20th century, along with some of the clinical applications of those theories. These theories include, for example, Distinctive Feature Theory, Generative Phonology, Natural Phonology, and various nonlinear theories, such as Feature Geometry. Clinicians need to have some understanding of phonological theory to make sound clinical decisions.

Descriptive Linguistics

Characteristics of Descriptive Linguistics

Descriptive Linguistics (also referred to as American Structuralism) was the predominant approach to phonology in the United States in the first part of the 20th century. Descriptive linguists were interested in precisely describing the *structural* aspects of languages (rather then their historical development). They were particularly interested in the **Amerindian** (Native American) **languages,** which differed greatly from the more familiar Indo-European languages, such as French, German, and Russian (e.g., see Bloomfield, 1933).

Clinical Applications of Descriptive Linguistics

The descriptive linguists' approach to phonology and sound systems, referred to as **phonemics,** focused on determining the phonemes used in a language.

Phonemes may be defined as the smallest units of sound that can change meaning. For example, in the word *cat,* there are three phonemes /k/, /æ/, and /t/, and in the word *pay,* there are two: /p/ and /e/. Note that it is the sounds that are important, not the letters. (See page 17 in Chapter 2.)

Variants of phonemes, called **allophones,** are also studied in phonemics. Allophones often occur in different word positions or phonetic contexts. For example, English voiceless stops /p/, /t/, and /k/ are produced with aspiration in word-initial position or preceding a stressed vowel, as in *pill,* but they are produced without aspiration (unaspirated) following an /s/ in a consonant cluster, as in *spill.* Phonemes and allophones are transcribed using phonetic transcription. In a narrow phonetic transcription, allophones are transcribed differently. In this example, the aspirated /p/ in *pill* would be transcribed as [pʰ], and the unaspirated /p/ in *spill* would be transcribed as [p⁼]. (Diacritical marks are described in more detail on page 20 in Chapter 2.)

Before about 1970, speech-language pathologists used a "sound-by-sound" approach to remediation in which each sound was dealt with as a separate entity. Although the term phoneme was sometimes used, a phonemic analysis was not necessarily performed. In fact, phonemics has never been widely applied in dealing with speech sound disorders in children. The principles and methods of phonemic analysis may be followed, however, if a clinician wishes to determine whether or not sounds are being used contrastively (i.e., to change meaning). For example, if a child says [be] for both *pay* and *bay,* that child is *not* using /p/ and /b/ contrastively. Rather, there is **neutralization** (or merging) of the adult English /p/–/b/ phonemic contrast. In this case, [be] is a **homonym**—one phonetic form representing two different words.

Behaviorist Theories

Some models of speech sound acquisition proposed in the middle part of the 20th century were based on behaviorist theories of psychology, which include Autism Theory and Ease of Perception Theory. Although linguists did not consider these to be acceptable models of children's phonological acquisition, they are discussed briefly here because of the influence of behaviorism on clinical practice.

Autism Theory

Mowrer's (1952, 1960) **Autism Theory** of speech sound acquisition (based on evidence from talking birds) emphasizes the emotional relationship between the "caregiver" and the "learner," as well as the role of reinforcement (Ferguson & Garnica, 1975). According to Mowrer, the learner's vocalizations themselves become reinforcing when they resemble those of the caregiver. Moreover, sounds that are similar to those of the caregiver are **selectively reinforced** by the caregiver, whereas others are not reinforced and therefore drop out. In this way, the learner's productions gradually become more like those of the caregiver. (These claims have not been supported by research, however.) This is a theory of **speech** sound acquisition because **phonological** acquisition involves much more than just learning to produce speech sounds (as discussed in Chapter 2).

Ease of Perception Theory

Olmsted's (1966) extension of Mowrer's (1952, 1960) theory is sometimes called the **Ease of Perception Theory** because it focuses on the importance of input and the perceptibility of sounds. It predicts that "easily discriminable" sounds will be learned first. Olmsted's theory had some support from two studies of actual children (e.g., Olmsted, 1971), but overall, his order of discriminability has not been well supported in the literature.

Clinical Applications

Behaviorist theories have had an important impact on the practice of speech-language pathology (e.g., see Winitz, 1969). For example, a stimulus-response (S-R) paradigm has often been used to change behavior. The client is provided with a **stimulus,** such as a model of the word *key,* and is expected to produce *key* with a correct initial /k/, the desired **response. Positive reinforcement,** such as praise or a small token, is provided on a schedule to increase the likelihood of that response occurring again. In some cases, sounds that cannot be elicited are "shaped" from similar sounds.

Universal Order Theory

Roman Jakobson

Jakobson (first syllable pronounced: /jɑ/) was a prolific European linguist in the structuralist tradition. As a member of the "Prague School" in the 1920s and 30s, he was interested in the concept of **opposition** or **distinctiveness** among sounds, as well as the idea of breaking phonemes down further into their distinctive phonetic properties or features.

Jakobson (1941/1968) believed that the same principles that account for phoneme inventories of adult languages also account for a child's acquisition of phonemic contrasts and the loss of such contrasts in aphasia. Specifically, the phonemic contrasts that are most common in languages of the world would be acquired earliest by children and would be most resistant to loss in aphasia. Conversely, phonemes that are rare in languages would be acquired later by children and would be lost earlier in aphasia.

The Principle of Maximal Contrast

Jakobson (1941/1968) attempted to account for the structure of phoneme inventories by what he called the **principle of maximal contrast.** This principle accounts for the basic consonant and vowel contrasts in a language. The most basic contrast in the sound system involves a totally closed vocal tract (as in the production of a stop consonant, such as /p/) and a maximally open vocal tract (as in the production of an open [low] vowel, such as /ɑ/). The next most basic opposition is a contrast between an oral consonant, such as /p/, and a nasal consonant, such as /m/. The first contrast in place of articulation involves a labial versus an alveolar consonant (e.g., /p/ versus /t/). The first vowel contrast involves a low versus a high vowel (/ɑ/ versus /i/). This is followed by a contrast between a high, front, unrounded vowel /i/ and a high, back, rounded vowel /u/. These contrasts mark the limits of the vowel space and result in a basic three-vowel system /ɑ, i, u/, which occurs, for example, in some of the native languages of Australia (Ladefoged, 2001).

Implicational Universals

Whereas the principle of maximal contrast is said to account for the basic consonant and vowel contrasts, Jakobson's (1941/1968) **implicational universals** (or laws of irreversible solidarity) account for additional facts about phoneme inventories. For instance, the implicational universal **back ⊃ front** (read as: "back implies front") predicts that if a language has back consonants, it will also have front consonants. Similarly, **fricatives ⊃ stops** ("fricatives imply stops") means that if a language has fricatives, it will also have stops. Because these laws are irreversible, we would not expect a language to have back consonants without front consonants or fricatives without stops.

These implicational universals also predict that in language acquisition, the implied member (on the right of the ⊃ symbol) should be acquired before the implying member (on the left of the ⊃). Moreover, the member on the right should also substitute for the one on the left. For example, /t/ (a front consonant) should be acquired before /k/ (a back consonant), and /t/ should also substitute for /k/. In language loss in aphasia, /k/ should be lost before /t/, etc. Because the principle of maximal contrast and the implicational universals govern children's acquisition of phonemic oppositions, the order of acquisition should be the same the world over **(universal).** This is the basis of Jakobson's (1941/1968) **Universal Order Theory.**

The Discontinuity View

In Jakobson's (1941/1968) view, **prelinguistic** (nonmeaningful) vocalization, such as babbling, is totally separate from (i.e., not related to) meaningful speech. This is sometimes referred to as the **discontinuity view.** Jakobson even went so far as to talk about a "silent period" between the two types of vocal behavior ("strict discontinuity").

Some Strengths and Weaknesses of the Universal Order Theory

Some aspects of Jakobson's (1941/1968) theory have held up quite well over time, such as the importance of front consonants and stop consonants in languages of the world and in children's acquisition. Other aspects, however, have been criticized as being overly simplistic or incorrect. For example, although some types of sounds (e.g., front stops and front nasals) tend to be acquired relatively early, and others (e.g., affricates and liquids) tend to be acquired later, most research has not supported the idea of a universal order of acquisition. In addition, Jakobson's discontinuity view has not been well supported by research on the transition from babbling to meaningful speech. In spite of its shortcomings, Jakobson's theory was very important in establishing phonological acquisition as a rich area of investigation.

Distinctive Feature Theory

Some Characteristics of Distinctive Feature Theory

Jakobson, like other members of the Prague School, was also interested in breaking phonemes down into their "distinctive phonetic properties" or "features." This became the basis for **Distinctive Feature Theory.** Jakobson and his colleagues wanted to find a small set of features (12–15) that could not be broken down further and that would be universal, accounting for significant contrasts in all spoken languages. They also wanted these features to be **binary,** meaning that each phonetic property was either present (+) or absent (–) (Jakobson, 1949). In addition, each phoneme in a language should be unique, differing from every other phoneme by at least one feature. For instance, /p/ and /b/ differ only in the value of the [voice] feature. Several sets of features were subsequently proposed (e.g., Jakobson, Fant, & Halle, 1952; Jakobson & Halle, 1956), but the set most widely used in speech-language pathology is essentially the one by Chomsky and Halle (1968).

Uses of Distinctive Features

Distinctive features are used to classify and describe the phonemes of a language. They also specify **natural phoneme classes** that share phonetic properties, such as stridency, and that undergo the same sound changes. To illustrate, the feature [+ nasal] specifies the natural class made up of the nasal consonants /m, n, ŋ/ in English. In general, it is not necessary to specify all of the features that comprise a sound. Those that can be predicted or inferred from other features are considered to be redundant; they can be "filled in" by what are called **redundancy rules.** For instance, phonemes that are [+ nasal] are also [+ sonorant], [+ voice], etc., but these features do not have to be mentioned, because they can be predicted from what we know about nasals. Distinctive features are also used in writing phonological rules, as discussed later in this chapter.

Markedness

Markedness is a complex concept that has been viewed in different ways by different phonologists. In Distinctive Feature Theory, a marked sound is basically one that has an added property as compared to another sound. For instance, /d/ is "marked" for voicing, relative to /t/. Markedness may be thought of as the opposite of naturalness. "Marked" sounds, sound classes, syllable structures, etc., are acquired later by children. On the other hand, "unmarked" or "natural" sounds, sound classes, etc., are more widespread in human languages and are acquired earlier by children. (See the discussion of Natural Phonology on pages 158–160.)

Clinical Applications of Distinctive Features

The first attempts to apply Distinctive Feature Theory in analyzing and remediating children's sound errors date back to the late 1960s and early 1970s. Early studies include those by Menyuk (1968), McReynolds and Huston (1971), Singh and Frank (1972), and Pollack and Rees (1972). (See summaries in Edwards & Shriberg, 1983.)

A detailed analysis procedure based on distinctive features was published by McReynolds and Engmann (1975). This procedure involves finding commonalities in the feature errors that underlie children's sound substitutions. Error percentages are then derived for each feature value (+ and –), across all phonemes. To illustrate, if a child says [bɪg] for *pig,* [do] for *toe,* [di] for *key,* etc., all of these substitution errors can be seen as involving the [– voice] feature ("minus voicing") in word-initial position. If this feature is incorrect a high percentage of the time across phonemes, it may be chosen for remediation. To remediate this feature error, target sounds are selected in which only this one feature is incorrect. In this example, /t/ and /p/, which are [– voice], would be contrasted with their minimally different [+ voice] counterparts /d/ and /b/ in minimal pairs, such as /ti/ versus /di/, /pe/ versus /be/, etc. (Note that /k/ would not be selected as a target sound in this case, because its substitute [d] differs in place of articulation, as well as voicing.) This approach of contrasting sounds that differ by just one feature (minimal pairs) is still widely used in treating phonological disorders. (See pages 81–82 in Chapter 5 for a summary.)

One limitation to the application of Distinctive Feature Theory is that only **substitution errors** can be handled satisfactorily—that is, errors in which one phoneme of English replaces another, as in [b] for /p/ or [d] for /s/. By definition, distortions are in the same phoneme category as the intended sound and therefore do not differ from it in distinctive features (e.g., an interdental /s/ has the same distinctive feature specification as a phonetically correct /s/). In omission errors, *all* the features of the intended sound are omitted. Perhaps because of these limitations, distinctive feature analysis never became the predominant approach in clinical phonology. Nonetheless, having a "working knowledge" of features is important because terms and concepts related to distinctive features are embedded in many phonological approaches.

Generative Phonology

A major phonological theory of the 20th century was Generative Phonology, described most fully by Chomsky and Halle in 1968. Their version of Generative Phonology is often referred to as Standard Generative Phonology (SGP). Only the basics of this complex theory are covered in this section. Two concepts from SGP have been influential in clinical phonology: phonological rules in the early 1970s, and underlying representations in the 1980s. Each is discussed here.

Phonological Rules and Applications

A **phonological rule** is a way of "capturing" or showing a sound change (e.g., a sound production error), such as when a child inappropriately applies voicing to an initial consonant (as in [bi] for *pea* and [du] for *two)* or fronts velars to alveolars (as in [ti] for *key* and [do] for *go).* Phonological rules are of primary importance in SGP. These rules account for **surface representations** (i.e., produced forms) that are derived from more abstract underlying representations. **Underlying representations** (URs) are the hypothesized mental representations of words to which phonological rules apply. URs are more abstract than produced forms, in part because related words that differ somewhat on the surface (when they are produced) are derived from the same UR. For example, the UR of both *public* and *publicity* would be /pʌblɪk/. When /ɪti/ is added to /pʌblɪk/, the /k/ becomes [s] by a rule called "velar softening," and the stress (emphasis) is shifted to the syllable preceding /ɪti/, creating the surface representation (the produced form) "publicity."

Writing Phonological Rules

In Generative Phonology, phonological rules have specific notations. To show how phonological rules are written, a sound change that is common in young children will be used as an example. This sound change involves replacing *voiced* sounds at the end of a word (i.e., in word-final position) with **voiceless** sounds. It is referred to as final consonant devoicing. Examples include [nos] for *nose,* [petʃ] for *page,* and [mæt] for *mad.* The rule showing this sound change can be written "formally" (using distinctive feature notation) as follows:

[– sonorant] → [– voice] / __ #

This rule states that sounds classified as [– sonorant] (i.e., obstruents: fricatives, affricates, and stops) become [– voice] (i.e., they are devoiced) when they occur at the end of the word, or literally, when preceding a word boundary (#).

In phonological rules, the arrow (→) always represents change and is read as "becomes" or "is replaced by." Whatever is to the left of the arrow is the **input** or the sound or sound class that is changed. Immediately to the right of the arrow is the **output;** this is the sound or sound class that results from the change. When a sound change takes place only in a particular position or context, as in word-final devoicing, the relevant context is shown after a slash. The context written as __#, as in our final devoicing example above, means literally "preceding a word boundary," and is interpreted as "in word-final position." (Word "boundaries" occur at the beginning and end of each word. The # symbol represents a word boundary. So, #__ would mean "following a word boundary" or "in word-initial position.") If a sound change takes place only in specific positions or contexts, as in our example, it is said to be **context sensitive.** On the other hand, a **context-free** sound change takes place without regard to context; no context is shown in the rule. A rule written as [– sonorant] → [– voice] indicates that obstruents are devoiced everywhere, across all positions.

In a **deletion rule,** a null symbol (ø) appears to the right of the arrow. That is, the feature or feature combination specified in the input becomes "nothing" or is deleted. An example is deletion of word-final consonants, which is written as:

[+ consonantal] → ø / __#

This rule indicates that consonant sounds are deleted when preceding a word boundary (/ __#), which is the word-final position.

An **addition** or insertion rule has a null sign to the left of the arrow, and the sound that is added appears after the arrow (e.g., ø → ə). For example, a child may insert a vowel between two consonants in a cluster, as in [bəlu] for blue. The formal rules of Generative Phonology are written with distinctive features; and there are many conventions regarding how they apply and how they are interpreted.

Clinical Applications of Phonological Rules

Beginning in 1970, several articles were published in which phonological rules were used to analyze the sound errors of children with multiple misarticulations (e.g., Compton, 1970; Lorentz, 1974; Oller, 1973). Investigators like these showed that phonological rules could help them observe and describe patterns in children's speech sound errors that would not be evident in a sound-by-sound approach. Formal phonological rules written in distinctive feature notation were never widely applied clinically, but one assessment procedure based on less formal rules was published later (Compton & Hutton, 1978). In addition, informal rules are often used as part of a more extensive phonological analysis to show specific sound changes that can later be combined and described in terms of phonological "processes" (e.g., Edwards, 1994).

Underlying Representations

As mentioned earlier, **underlying representations** (URs) are the hypothesized mental representations of words to which phonological rules apply. Generative phonologists did not always agree as to how abstract URs should be (that is, how far removed and different from the actual produced forms). In any case, all related surface forms had to be derived from a common UR by phonological rules. For example, in order to derive both *electric* and *electricity* from a common UR, generative phonologists proposed the UR of *electricity* to be /ɛlɛktrɪk + ɪti/. The rule of velar softening then changes the /k/ to [s] preceding the *-ity* suffix.

Child phonologists have generally assumed that children's underlying representations are like the broad adult forms. Dinnsen, Elbert, and Weismer (1979, 1980), however, argued that children with speech sound disorders may have **unique** underlying representations, and that this has to be established for each individual child. To illustrate, Dinnsen and his colleagues discussed two children with phonological disorders, neither of whom produced final consonants. Jamie, age 7:2, omitted final stops, as in [dɔ:] for *dog,* but when the diminutive ending /i/ was added, the stop showed up, as in [dɔdi]. Dinnsen et al. interpreted this as evidence for an adult-like UR (/dɔg/), along with a final consonant deletion rule. For Matthew, age 3:11, however, the stops did *not* show up when the diminutive ending was added. So *dog* was [dɑ], and *doggie* was [dɑi]. Because Matthew gave no evidence of "knowing" about final consonants, his UR for *dog* was said to be like his produced form /dɑ/. (One point on which this work has been criticized is the considerable age discrepancy between these two children, 7:2 versus 3:11.)

Productive Phonological Knowledge

Elbert and Gierut (1986) incorporated the concept of underlying representations into the broader concept of productive phonological knowledge, which is said to include all the information that is stored mentally for each morpheme. Results of a set of detailed analyses are used to "rank" the child's phonological knowledge on a continuum of six **knowledge types,** from the most knowledge (type 1) to the least knowledge (type 6). Sounds with type 1 knowledge are always produced correctly, and are not affected by phonological rules; their underlying representations are said to be "adult-like." In contrast, sounds with type 6 knowledge are *never* produced correctly and are not present in the child's inventory; their underlying representations are said to be "nonadult-like." For Elbert and Gierut (1986), the child's URs are generally considered to be the same as his or her produced forms unless **morphophonemic alternation** is observed, as in the *dog–doggie* example. (It is important to note that this approach relies on production evidence, in spite of the fact that URs are mental representations that cannot be directly observed.)

Clinical Applications of Productive Phonological Knowledge

Elbert and Gierut (1986) hypothesized that differences in productive phonological knowledge might account for differences in children's abilities to generalize remediation improvements to sounds that have not specifically been targeted. Gierut's (1989, 1990, 1992) research supports the view that children with speech sound disorders generalize more extensively (e.g., add more new sounds to their repertoire) when they are first taught sounds for which they have "least phonological knowledge" (knowledge type 6). Independent support for this approach has not been reported, however, and the findings of Rvachew and Nowak (2001) did not support the contention.

Natural Phonology

Natural Phonological Processes

The phonological theory that has had the greatest impact in the field of speech-language pathology is Stampe's **Natural Phonology** (1969, 1972, 1973). (See also Donegan & Stampe, 1979.) According to Stampe, children are born with an innate system of phonetically motivated **natural phonological processes,** such as stopping of fricatives (as in s → t, f → p), fronting of velars (as in k → t, g → d), and simplification of consonant clusters (as in sp → p, br → b), etc. These processes are said to be "phonetically motivated" or "motivated by the physical properties of speech." Their purpose is "to maximize the perceptual characteristics of speech and minimize its articulatory difficulties" (Stampe, 1972, p. 9). For example, consonant clusters (such as str) are more difficult to produce than are single consonants (such as s, t, r); this is the basis for the natural process referred to as cluster reduction or cluster simplification. Stampe makes a distinction between natural processes, which are innate, and rules, which are learned and language-specific (e.g., rules for forming noun plurals in English). Natural processes are said to show up in dialect variation and historical language change, as well as phonological acquisition.

Stampe's View of Children's Underlying Representations

In Stampe's (1969, 1972, 1973) Natural Phonology Theory, the underlying representations to which natural processes apply are basically the same as the broad adult forms. To illustrate, whether the word *train* is produced as [teɪn], [deɪ], or [tweɪn], the child's underlying representation is taken to be /treɪn/.

Stampe's view of the child's phonological system is very simple. It consists of the child's underlying representations and a set of natural phonological processes that apply, resulting in the child's surface representations:

Child's Underlying Representations (broad adult forms)	→	Natural Phonological Processes	→	Child's Surface Representations (produced forms)

To illustrate, if a child says [din] for *green,* it is assumed that the UR is the broad adult form /grin/. Liquid cluster reduction (eliminating the difficult liquid part of the cluster) and velar fronting (fronting the velar stop to an easier alveolar stop) both apply. (In this example, liquid cluster reduction and velar fronting are **constituent** or **interacting processes.)**

Innate Phonological System Revisions

Early in a child's phonological development, natural processes are said to apply whenever and wherever they can. As the child matures, the innate phonological system changes by means of three mechanisms, which Stampe (1969, 1972, 1973) refers to as limitation, ordering, and suppression.

Limitation refers to the fact that over time, processes may apply to fewer segments and/or in fewer environments. For instance, a child may at first delete **all** final consonants, but later on delete only final **stops.** Similarly, different children may limit processes differently, resulting in some of the variation observed in phonological acquisition.

In **ordering,** processes are sequenced such that one cannot apply after the other. For example, if a child's voicing process cannot apply after (and to the output of) cluster reduction, the child will say [bɪn] for *pin* (with just voicing), while at the same time saying [pɪn] for *spin* (with just cluster reduction). In Stampe's view, such seeming "inconsistencies" show that phonological processes are not motorically based. (In this example, the child can produce initial [p], but only when it represents an /sp/ cluster.)

When a process is **suppressed,** it no longer applies at all. Grunwell (1982, 1987) presented a **process chronology** summarizing the **ages of suppression** for a number of common phonological processes (see Table 3.3, on page 36). These are the ages at which the processes are no longer evident in the speech of children with typical development. One goal of remediation based on Stampe's model is to help the child eliminate age-inappropriate phonological processes.

Clinical Applications of Natural Phonology

The first clinical studies using a phonological process approach (i.e., based on natural phonology) were conducted in the early 1970s, shortly after the first clinical applications of distinctive features and phonological rules. (In fact, clinical phonology can be thought of as beginning in about 1970.) Early clinical applications of phonological processes include those of Edwards and Bernhardt (1973a, 1973b), Grunwell (1975), Ingram (1976), and Oller (1973). These researchers showed that phonological processes could be used to describe the patterns evident in children's sound errors and to consequently develop remediation goals based on those descriptions.

Phonological process/pattern approaches are still widely used in both assessing and remediating speech sound disorders. A frequent goal of remediation is to help children suppress inappropriate phonological processes (Tyler, Edwards, & Saxman, 1987) or acquire new phonological patterns, that will negate the effects of the child's phonological deviations (e.g., Hodson & Paden, 1983, 1991). Interacting deviations may be remediated separately so that the child has to change just one feature (such as voicing or stridency) at a time (Edwards, 1992; Kelman & Edwards, 1994).

Prosodic Theory

Characteristics of Prosodic Theory

Waterson's (1970, 1971) **Prosodic Theory** of phonological acquisition emphasizes the importance of perception and input (Menn, 1976) and states that because of the uniqueness of each child's input, the resulting patterns of acquisition are also unique. The Prosodic Theory is a "nonsegmental" theory because the basic unit is considered to be the whole word rather than the **phoneme**. According to Waterson, the child perceives similarities among adult words that share certain salient features (e.g., nasality or frication) and uses them to form "structural patterns," which then form the basis for the child's productions. To illustrate, one of several "structural patterns" used by Waterson's (1971) son was a "sibilant structure." It was used for several monosyllabic words that contained voiceless sibilants in final position, such as *fish, dish, vest, fetch.* He produced all of these words with a high lax vowel and a final palatal sibilant, as in [ɪʃ] or [ʊʃ] for *fish,* [ʊʃ] for *vest,* [dɪʃ] for *dish,* etc. Using examples from her son, Waterson (1970) showed how the child's productions change over time as perception improves and structural patterns are revised.

Clinical Applications of Prosodic Theory

Although there are some appealing aspects to Waterson's (1970, 1971) Prosodic Theory, such as the fact that it can account for differences between children and within one child, it is limited, focusing on very early acquisition (under 2 years of age). There is much that it does not account for. For example, it does not consider phonemes and does not attempt to account for general patterns of acquisition. (See Ferguson & Garnica, 1975, for a more detailed discussion.) Prosodic Theory has not been applied clinically; it is included here because it foreshadows the later nonlinear theories.

Interactionist-Discovery Theory

Interactionist-Discovery Theory, or the **Cognitive Theory,** was developed in the mid-1970s to account for phonological acquisition in children. Menn (1976) and Kiparsky and Menn (1977) most fully articulated the theory, although some tenets of it were expressed earlier, for example by Ingram (1974a, 1974b), and Ferguson and Farwell (1975). (See also Ferguson & Macken, 1980; Macken & Ferguson, 1983; and Menn, 1978, 1980.)

A Discovery-Oriented Approach

The Interactionist-Discovery Theory is considered a discovery-oriented approach because it stresses the active organization and creativity of the child. Children are said to form and test hypotheses about their language. They organize distinctions into manageable pieces and "discover" the structure of the language.

In this view, rules connect the child's perceived forms to his or her produced forms. There are no innate processes; rather, children invent their own phonological rules by "active experimentation" and the use of strategies.

Children Limiting Their Output

According to Menn (1976), the child masters "special cases" (p. 169) and tries to find patterns to relate them; these patterns are then generalized to new words. Further, children may "exploit" their capabilities by adding new words that are similar to those already in their lexicon, for example, because they contain labials or nasals. Vihman (1981) also noted such "selection." Menn argued that young children may limit the variety of their output by "consolidating" similar outputs or using a few set patterns (compare Waterson, 1970, 1971).

Clinical Applications of Interactionist-Discovery Theory

This theory has had more of an impact on studies of typical phonological acquisition than on clinical research or practice. While Stampe's (1969, 1972, 1973) Natural Phonology Theory accounts well for similarities among children and for general patterns, the Interactionist-Discovery Theory accounts well for individual differences. It appears to be particularly applicable to very early acquisition, when each word seems to follow its own developmental path, and phonological acquisition is closely tied to the acquisition of words. Early studies that take this more cognitive perspective include those of Fey and Gandour (1982), Klein (1981), Leonard, Newhoff, and Mesalam (1980), and Vihman (1976).

Nonlinear Theories

Characteristics of Nonlinear Theories

Since the late 1970s, a number of theories have been proposed that, as a group, are referred to as **nonlinear** or **multilinear. Linear** theories (like those we have discussed so far) focus mainly on strings of **segments** (consonants and vowels) on one level. In contrast, nonlinear theories are concerned with **hierarchical relationships** among linguistic units (e.g., segments, syllables, words) that occur on different levels or tiers. These levels are often shown in branching tree diagrams such as the one in Figure 9.1. Prosodic (stress) information is included, in addition to segmental information. This section provides an overview of a few nonlinear theories.

Figure 9.1 *Metrical Phonology Representation of the Word* Blanket

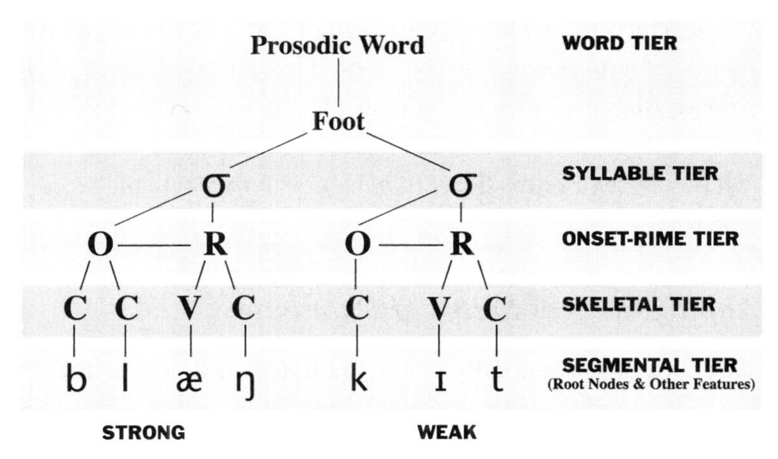

Source: Bernhardt & Stoel-Gammon (1994)

Metrical Phonology

Metrical Phonology is a nonlinear theory that focuses on **syllable structure** and **prosodic features** such as stress and tone. To illustrate, the syllable structure of the word *blanket* is shown schematically in Figure 9.1. The **word tier** is the highest level.

Blanket is a **prosodic word** because it contains just one primary (or main) stress, which occurs on the first syllable. It also consists of one **foot**—a metrical unit comprised of a **strong** (stressed) and a **weak** (unstressed) **syllable,** as shown on the **syllable tier** (the sigma symbol /σ/ represents a syllable). Because the strong syllable (S) occurs to the left of the weak syllable (w), it is a **trochaic** foot **(Sw).** If the stronger syllable occurred on the right, as in *giraffe,* it would be an iambic foot **(wS).** (English is said to have a "trochaic bias" because most of our two-syllable words are "left-prominent.")

Each syllable is made up of two parts, the **onset** (O) and the **rime** (R)**.** The syllable tier "dominates" the O-R tier. The **onset** of a syllable consists of any consonants (up to three in English, such as /skw/ and /str/) that precede the vowel—referred to as the nucleus. The **rime** contains the nucleus and any consonants following it (the **coda).** The only essential part of a syllable is the **nucleus** (the loudest part, which is also referred to as the peak; it is usually a vowel). *Eye* [aɪ] is an example of a **monosyllabic** (one-syllable) word with just a nucleus, and *tea* [ti] is a monosyllabic word with no coda. The consonant and vowel composition of each syllable is shown on the **skeletal tier,** and the segments that fill each slot are shown on the **segmental tier.** So, *blanket* is a two-syllable word made up of one trochaic foot.

Clinical Applications of Metrical Phonology

Clinical studies done at least partially within the framework of metrical phonology include those of Bernhardt and Gilbert (1992), and Vellemann and Shriberg (1999; see also Schwartz, 1992). Bernhardt and Stemberger (2000) presented an analysis approach that includes analyzing a child's syllables and stress patterns, as well as the types of sounds that can occur in each syllable position for the child. (For example, a child might produce only nasals in coda position.) Bernhardt and Stemberger integrated such information into their suggestions for remediation. For example, they targeted both syllable structures and segments, with new sounds being remediated in existing syllable structures, and existing sounds being used in new syllable structures.

Feature Geometry

Feature Geometry (Sagey, 1986) is a nonlinear theory that focuses on the features that comprise segments. In feature geometry, unlike Distinctive Feature Theory, features are organized into **hierarchies,** with some features "dominating" others, and features with similar functions (e.g., place features) grouped together. The skeletal tier contains C (consonant) and V (vowel) "nodes," as was shown in Figure 9.1. Each C or V dominates a **root node** that specifies the feature content of that segment (Chin & Dinnsen, 1991).

Segments Representation in Feature Geometry

Sagey's (1986) representation of the feature geometry for an English consonant (C) is shown in Figure 9.2. Each root node dominates two **binary** (+/–) feature

Figure 9.2 *Sagey's Feature Geometry for English Consonants*

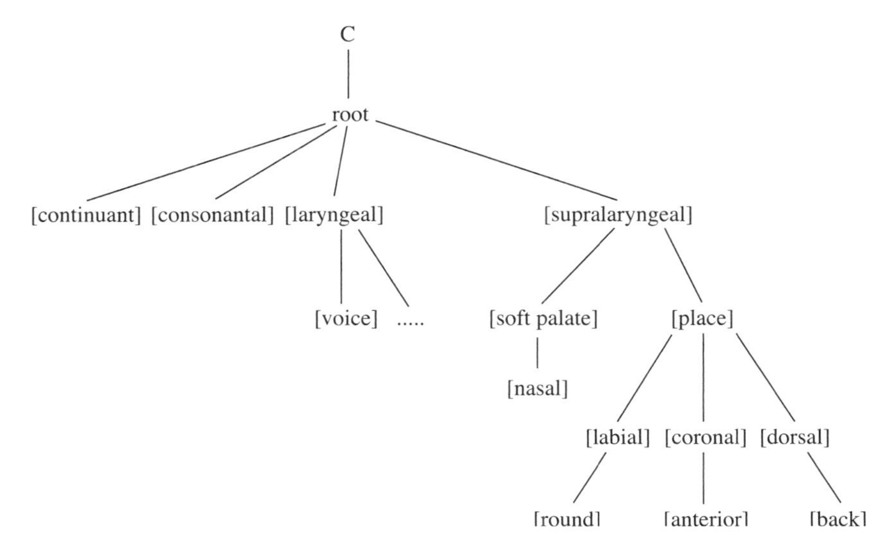

Source: Sagey (1986)

nodes: **[continuant]** and **[consonantal].** This means that each consonant is either [+ continuant] or [– continuant] and either [+ consonantal] or [– consonantal]. Each root node also dominates two "class nodes:" [laryngeal] and [supralaryngeal]. The **[laryngeal]** node dominates features having to do with voicing, such as +/– [voice], and the **[supralaryngeal]** node dominates **[soft palate]** (for +/– **[nasal]),** and **[place]** for the "articulator nodes" **[labial], [coronal],** and **[dorsal].** Each articulator node, in turn, dominates additional binary features, such as [round], [anterior], and [back] that specify how the articulator is used. To give an example, /n/ would be classified as [– continuant], [+ consonantal], [+ voice], [+ nasal], and [+ anterior]. The continuants /s/ and /ʃ/ would be the same in all features except [anterior], with /s/ being [+ anterior] and /ʃ/ being [– anterior] because /ʃ/ is produced further back in the mouth than /s/.

Clinical Applications of Feature Geometry

Chin and Dinnsen (1991) described the clinical application of Feature Geometry. These phonologists focused on the processes of assimilation and coalescence, arguing that Feature Geometry provides a better explanation for these phenomena than other theories. **Assimilation** is shown to involve **feature spreading** from one segment to another, as in [gɔg] for *dog,* with spreading of the [dorsal] feature from the coda /g/ to the onset /d/. Segment **coalescence,** as in [fɪm] for *swim,* is accounted for by **reassociation** of the [labial] feature of the second consonant /w/ with the supralaryngeal node of /s/, resulting in the voiceless labial continuant [f].

Optimality Theory

Characteristics of Optimality Theory

The basic units of **Optimality Theory (OT)** are **constraints** (McCarthy & Prince, 1995). **Output constraints** (also referred to as well-formedness or markedness constraints) capture limitations on what can be pronounced (the output). In contrast, **faithfulness constraints** require faithfulness to the input by prohibiting addition and deletion and requiring features to be "preserved." Like most phonological theories, OT was developed to account for adult languages, but the examples given here were selected for their relevance to children's phonologies. For example, the output constraint written as **Syl>Onset,** or just **Onset,** is interpreted as "syllables must have an onset," and the constraint written as **Complex(Onset),** or ***Complex(Onset),** means "onsets cannot be complex;" that is, clusters are prohibited in syllable onsets. Examples of other constraints that might be written to capture limitations on children's productions are listed below, with brief interpretations. Because there are different ways of formulating constraints, alternate versions are given.

Examples of output constraints:

*Coda = Not(Coda) = "Consonants cannot occur in coda position."

*Strident = Not(Strident) = "No stridents are produced."

*Sequence([dorsal]...[coronal]) = "No velar-alveolar sequences are produced."

Examples of faithfulness constraints:

MAX = "Segments cannot be deleted."

DEP = "Segments cannot be inserted."

IDENT-VOICE = "The voicing feature (+ or –) is preserved."

IDENT (Dorsal) = "The dorsal (back) feature is maintained."

Constraints and Ranking

Constraints are assumed to be part of **Universal Grammar (UG),** that is, innate and universal to all languages (Barlow & Gierut, 1999, p. 1485). Variation across languages, as well as variation among children (or in one child over time), is accounted for by the **relative ranking** of constraints. For example, **NotComplex** or ***Complex** (which prohibits clusters) must be ranked low in English, because English has many consonant clusters. In a language with few or no clusters, this constraint would be ranked high. Similarly, early in development, when a child is producing no clusters, ***Complex** would be ranked high in that child's phonology, but later on, when the child is able to produce clusters, ***Complex** would be ranked lower. Relative ranking of constraints is shown by a double arrow. For example, ***Complex>>MAX** means that ***Complex** is ranked higher than **MAX.** Lower ranked constraints are less important and more likely to be "violated" than higher ranked constraints.

Constraint Table

Possible productions of a word, along with the relevant constraints, are shown in a **constraint table** or **tableau,** as in Table 9.1, on page 168. **Violations** of constraints are shown with an asterisk (*), and a **fatal violation** (one involving a highly ranked constraint) is shown by an asterisk plus an exclamation point (*!). The production or "candidate" whose ranking violates the **least** important constraints is the "optimal" one, shown by the **manual indicator** (the pointing finger). Four possible productions of the word *snake* are shown in Table 9.1 (based on Barlow & Gierut, 1999). The first possibility, [sneɪk], is ruled out because it contains a cluster and therefore violates the highest ranked constraint (a "fatal violation"). The optimal rendition is [neɪk] because it violates just one constraint that is ranked fairly low (the segment /s/ is deleted in violation of the MAX constraint).

As a child matures, **re-ranking** of constraints occurs. Specifically, output constraints are "demoted," and faithfulness constraints are "promoted" so that the

Table 9.1 *An Optimality Theory Constraint Table*
"snake" /sneɪk/ → [neɪk]

/sneɪk/	**Complex*	**s*	*Max*[1]	*Onset*[2]
sneɪk	*!	*		
eɪk			**!	*
seɪk		*!	*	
☞ neɪk			*	

1 "Max" prohibits deletion.
2 "Onset" means that all syllables must begin with a consonant (an "onset").

Source: Barlow & Gierut (1999)

child's output eventually "matches" the input (the adult form). A goal of intervention based on OT would be to facilitate re-ranking of a child's constraints.

Relationships of Phonological Processes and Constraints

In Optimality Theory (OT), phonological processes may be viewed as **repairs** for the child's output constraints (Bernhardt & Stemberger, 2000). To illustrate, if a child has the constraint ***Complex,** which prohibits clusters, liquid cluster reduction could "repair" words like *blue* and *plane* to make them pronounceable (as [bu], [peɪn]), and /s/ cluster reduction could make words like *snow* and *stove* pronounceable by deleting the /s/ ([no], [tov]). Bernhardt and Stemberger (2000) provide many such examples.

Clinical Applications of Optimality Theory

Clinical applications of Optimality Theory began to appear in the late 1990s. For example, both Barlow (2001) and Stemberger and Bernhardt (1997) presented case studies to illustrate the application of OT to specific children with phonological impairments. (See also Barlow, 2002; Barlow & Gierut, 1999; and Bernhardt & Stemberger, 2000). More research is needed regarding the applicability of OT for phonological analysis and intervention.

Gestural Phonology

Characteristics of Gestural Phonology

In **Gestural Phonology**—also referred to as Articulatory Phonology (e.g., Browman & Goldstein, 1992)—the phonological system is based on articulation, and phonological representations are described in terms of "articulatory organization" (Kent, 1997). The basic units of this theory are gestures. A **gesture** is defined as "an abstract characterization of an articulatory event" (Browman & Goldstein, 1992, p. 155) or as a "class of articulatory movements" (Kent, 1997, p. 253) involving, for example, the velum or the lips.

Gestural Score

A **gestural score** represents, on different levels or tiers, several movements (gestures) that may overlap in time. The gestures are organized to reflect the articulatory patterns of an utterance (Kent, 1997). For example, a gestural score would show velic closure on one level, lip closure on another level, and glottal opening on still another level. Because gestures are represented on separate levels or tiers (to capture their independence), it is possible to show their relative timing.

The tiers of a gestural score may also be shown in a tree diagram. In this case, velic articulations (concerning nasality) are on a separate tier from glottal function (e.g., voicing). A separate **oral tier** has branches for the lips, tongue tip, and tongue body. (These articulators are grouped together because they are all related to mandibular function and therefore are not totally independent.) The velic, glottal, and oral tiers are all related to the **skeletal tier,** which shows the syllable structure of the utterance (Kent, 1997). Other tiers include the **rhythmic tier** (for stress levels) and **functional tiers** that allow for overlap between consonants and vowels.

Relationship of Gestures and Phonological Processes

According to Kent (1997), phonetic changes such as the insertion or deletion of segments, assimilation, etc., may be accounted for by changes in the magnitude or phasing of gestures. For example, stopping may be described as an error in "scaling" or regulating the magnitude of an articulatory movement, in this case producing closure instead of close approximation of the articulators (Kent, 1997). Epenthesis (e.g., as in [bəlu] for *blue*) may be explained as involving errors in "intersyllabic phasing"; if the gestures for the adjacent consonants in a cluster do not overlap properly, an intrusive vowel (such as schwa) will occur.

Clinical Applications of Gestural Phonology

Gestural Phonology has not yet been applied in studies of children with phonological disorders. In her article concerning reading problems and the role of phonological awareness, however, Mody (2003) draws heavily on a gestural model. In addition, Kent (1997) describes a small number of studies that have applied this model to motor speech disorders such as dysarthria and apraxia (discussed more fully in Weismer, Tjaden, & Kent, 1995a, 1995b), and he points out the potential applicability to developmental phonological disorders. Gestural Phonology is appealing because of the close connection between the phonological system and articulation that is at the core of the theory. Further research is needed to explore its clinical potential.

Summary

Over the course of the past 30+ years, phonology has greatly expanded the range of options available for speech-language pathologists who assess and treat children with many misarticulations and reduced intelligibility. Instead of routinely using a sound-by-sound approach, in which error sounds are regarded as separate entities, it is now commonplace for clinicians to look for and treat patterns of errors. Exactly what those patterns are like and how they are described depends in part on the theory that one is following.

It is impossible to predict the future changes that will take place. It is likely, however, that as new theories of phonology are developed, at least some of them will lead to more insightful approaches that will further enhance the procedures available to clinicians who assess and remediate severe speech sound disorders in children.

CHAPTER 10

Major Clinical Phonology Issues, Concerns & Research Needs

Barbara Williams Hodson

It is not unusual for professions to have issues, controversies, and challenges as they grow and move forward. For example, the profession of education is notorious for its "reading wars," with pendulum swings between holistic "top down" methods (e.g., whole language) and a "bottom up" emphasis on teaching skills (e.g., phonics). Psychology is known for its "heated battles" (e.g., operant conditioning and strict behaviorism versus cognitive theories and principles). Speech-language pathology, which is considered to be a youngster compared to professions such as education and psychology, has its own set of issues. In the 1970s, the "hot button" issue in helping professions was **accountability,** with individualized education programs; the current "battle cry" is **evidence-based practice.** Clearly, professions such as speech-language pathology do need more well-designed experimental intervention studies.

Clinical phonology, which is the focus of this book, is one of the newer specialty areas within the speech-language pathology profession. We have our own issues and controversies, ranging from phoneme acquisition norms to oral-motor exercises. One of the most fundamental clinical phonology concerns pertains to severity.

Severity of Involvement

Severity of the client's speech sound disorder is a critical consideration for numerous aspects related to conducting research and making clinical decisions. Yet severity has been one of the most neglected aspects of clinical phonology. Some research reports do not include any specific information regarding preintervention severity levels. Other investigators provide the numbers of errors and/or percentile ranks based on standardized articulation tests (e.g., Goldman & Fristoe, 2000), but specific data are lacking regarding which or how many of the errors were omissions, substitutions, or distortions. Thus, it is not uncommon for children with quite different phonological systems to obtain similar scores on such measures. Over 30 years ago, Higgs (1970) pointed out that the "correct/incorrect" classification "hides a natural step by step development towards the 'correct' utterance which takes place over time" (p. 262). (For an example of this phenomenon, see Table 7.4, on page 121, for transcriptions of a client's productions over time.)

The most common method for designating severity currently reported in clinical research studies involves calculating the Percentage of Consonants Correct (PCC; Shriberg & Kwiatkowski, 1980). Velleman (2005) reported that one of her clients received the same PCC score at age 8 years that he had received at age 5 even though he was "vastly more intelligible" (p. 26). She validated this statement regarding the child's intelligibility gains when she showed videos of this client at ages 5 and 8 years at an ASHA Convention miniseminar (Flahive, Hodson, & Velleman, 2005). Velleman (2005) concluded "measures that rely on segmental accuracy alone, such as the PCC, may give an inappropriate view of the child's progress in therapy" (p. 26).

Shriberg, Austin, Lewis, McSweeny, and Wilson (1997) stated that the Percentage of Consonants Correct–Revised (PCC–R) is the "most appropriate metric for comparisons involving speakers of diverse speech status" and that it has "greater sensitivity to true involvement because of the focus on deletion and substitution errors" (p. 720). Nonetheless, most published clinical phonology studies report data from the PCC rather than the PCC–R. (The PCC–R does not score distortions as incorrect, but omissions and substitutions still receive equal weighting, whereas for the PCC, distortions, substitutions, and omissions are weighted the same.)

The determination of severity has been somewhat elusive (Flipsen, Hammer, & Yost, 2005; Gordon-Brannan & Hodson, 2000). Procedures range from listener ratings (e.g., Likert scales) of connected speech samples to word imitation (e.g., Morris, Wilcox, & Schooling, 1995) to calculating percentages of identifiable/ intelligible words. These methods have been found to be highly intercorrelated, but no one method alone, as yet, seems to be completely adequate. It may be that a formula needs to be derived that incorporates some combination of factors.

Clinical treatment studies need valid methods for specifying severity levels, and speech-language practitioners need appropriate determiners for individual clients to assist them in making evidence-based practice decisions. Clearly, incorporating a valid method for determining severity is an area of great need in clinical phonology.

Phoneme Acquisition Norms

A second area that has led to a great deal of confusion and consternation pertains to typical speech development norms. Early research focused on determining when individual phonemes were "mastered" (e.g., Poole, 1934; Prather, Hendrick, & Kern, 1975; Templin, 1957). Data from such normative studies, as well as more recent investigations (e.g., Smit, Hand, Freilinger, Bernthal, & Bird, 1990), have been used extensively for determining a child's eligibility for receiving services and also for selecting target sounds. A common practice in school settings has been that a sound is not to be targeted unless there is a delay of at least 1 year based on some published normative data. Table 10.1, on page 174, provides phoneme acquisition ages (based on studies published in 1934, 1957, 1975, and 1990) for the two sounds that are targeted most by SLPs: /s/ and /r/.

Table 10.1 *Acquisition Ages for Frequent Intervention Targets /s/ and /r/*

Researcher/Date	/s/	/r/
Poole (1934)	7:6	7:6
Templin (1957)	4:0	4:0
Prather et al. (1975)	3:8	3:4
Smit et al. (1990)	8:0	8:0

Sources: Poole (1934); Prather et al. (1975); Smit et al. (1990); Templin (1957)

Some of the discrepancies are related to the differences in methods used to obtain samples, the words used, and the criteria set (e.g., percentage required) for acquisition (Smit, 1986). Another issue pertains to whether a totally correct/incorrect dichotomous scoring was used and if there were any allowances for allophonic variations (e.g., distortions) or regional dialect differences.

Discrepancies such as those shown in Table 10.1 have led to inconsistencies in service delivery from school district to school district (and even within school districts). Moreover, results of clinical phonology research studies may be influenced by the normative data selected. For example, Gierut, Morrisette, Hughes, and Rowland (1996) reported two single-subject design studies involving nine children in an ASHA journal article. In Study I, /r/ was listed as an "early acquired" sound (based on Templin's [1957] normative data); in Study II, /r/ was listed as a "later acquired" sound (using Smit et al. [1990] norms). Gierut and her colleagues reported that treatment of later-acquired phonemes (/v/, /ʤ/, /ð/ versus /l/, /k/, /r/ in Study I; /r/, /θ/, /s/ versus /k/, /g/, /f/ in Study II) led to greater "system-wide changes," but the discrepancy regarding /r/ was not explained.

Stimulability

Another aspect whose role in clinical decision-making research has had some controversy is stimulability. Stimulability testing is conducted to determine what sound(s) (e.g., /s/) or word structure(s) (e.g., /s/ cluster) not currently produced spontaneously by a child can be elicited with assistance from the clinician.

Elicitation efforts typically start with a model by the clinician followed by an imitative production by the child. Children who succeed at this level are considered to be "highly stimulable." If a child does not succeed, additional assists (e.g., tactile cues, amplification) are provided. The degree and type(s) of assistance required for eliciting an accurate production need to be documented. In some instances, however, a child cannot produce certain sounds (e.g., /k/, /r/) at the time of the stimulability testing. Such sounds are called "nonstimulable."

Some phonologists advocate targeting nonstimulable, later-acquired sounds first in intervention rather than stimulable sounds. Findings by Rvachew and Nowak (2001), based on a controlled experimental study involving 48 participants, however, were not in agreement. Children who targeted stimulable sounds in their study demonstrated greater gains than the children who targeted nonstimulable sounds.

Part of the issue may be related to the operational definition of stimulability. Historically, SLPs have waited to target a sound until it is stimulable because targeting/practicing a sound that the child cannot yet produce leads to reinforcement of the inaccurate kinesthetic image rather than to stimulability and generalization. It is not an uncommon practice, however, for a practitioner to spend a couple of minutes during intervention sessions enhancing stimulability of one or more sounds.

Childhood Apraxia of Speech

Childhood apraxia has been discussed extensively in the literature. A major symposium (Shriberg & Campbell, 2002) was planned to obtain consensus; however, the information contained in the proceedings of this conference indicated that there are many more questions than answers. The term currently preferred by the American Speech-Language-Hearing Association (ASHA) is "**suspected Childhood Apraxia of Speech (sCAS)**" because as yet there are no agreed-upon definitive criteria. Apraxia has frequently been an "umbrella term for children with persisting and serious speech difficulties in the absence of obvious causation, regardless of the precise nature of their unintelligibility" (Stackhouse, 1992, p. 30).

Commonly reported characteristics include the following:

- Motor planning/programming/sequencing problems
- Slower diadochokinetic rate
- Limited phonetic and phonotactic repertoires
- Reduplicated syllables
- Prosody/Suprasegmental differences
- Vowel deviations
- Inconsistencies
- A gap between receptive and expressive language/phonology abilities

Typically there has been an "either/or" dichotomy (e.g., apraxia versus phonology) when many (if not most) of the children whose phonological deviations place them in the profound category of phonological severity (Hodson, 2004) demonstrate the characteristics listed above.

One of the major concerns is an "overlabeling" of children. Moreover, instead of considering overlapping factors, there has been a tendency to discount or "rule out" other possible etiological factors (e.g., hearing) when co-occurring factors are often present. Another concern is that expectations for progress are often lowered for children with the sCAS label, and intervention goals typically exclude phonology. A common intervention practice for these children and others with speech sound disorders involves oral-motor exercises (Watson & Lof, 2005).

Oral-Motor Exercises

Oral-motor exercises are extremely popular in intervention sessions for children with speech sound disorders even if no known neuromuscular problems exist. Many anecdotal stories are available from advocates reporting success, but evidence-based research studies are lacking. Moreover, there are concerns regarding scientific and theoretical bases for oral-motor exercises. Lof (2003) reported that oral-motor exercises do not have an influence on the development of speech sounds. Forrest (2002) stated that "oral-motor exercises may be harmful by laying a framework of movement patterns that are contrary to those used in speech" (p. 22).

Phonological Intervention Research

Ingram (1986) and Kamhi (2005) have stated that all intervention methods are effective. A major issue, however, may be severity. It is likely that all intervention methods are similarly effective for children with mild/moderate levels of disorders. A question arises regarding effectiveness of various approaches for children at the other end of the continuum.

Most intervention programs are phoneme-oriented. The majority of these focus on mastering each phoneme before progressing to the next target. Some use contrastive techniques (e.g., minimal pairs, maximal oppositions, multiple oppositions). A few target word structures, referred to as "phonotactic" by Velleman (2002). Our preference for children with severe/profound disordered expressive phonological systems is to target patterns that are deficient, including word structures related to omissions (e.g., /s/ clusters, final consonants), as well as phoneme categories (e.g., velars, stridents). Phonemes are considered to be a means to an end, rather than the true targets.

There is a great need for large, well-designed controlled experimental studies comparing outcomes of various types of intervention (e.g., oral-motor, phoneme-oriented, phonological patterns) and various goals (e.g., vertical, horizontal, cyclical) and targets (e.g., singleton /f/ versus /s/ clusters) for children with highly unintelligible speech (severe/profound severity level of involvement). The number of children participating in each type of intervention needs to be large because children with speech sound disorders are extremely heterogeneous (e.g., Harbers, Paden, & Halle, 1999), and some confounding factors, such as capability and focus (see Shriberg, 1997), cannot be controlled. Clinician instruction and fidelity monitoring for the respective intervention approaches/goals would be crucial. Intervention goals and procedures and also contact hours would need to be documented carefully.

Summary

Some of the major issues and research needs in clinical phonology have been discussed in this chapter, including severity of involvement, phoneme acquisition norms, stimulability, childhood apraxia of speech, oral-motor exercises, and phonological intervention research. This list certainly is not meant to be all inclusive, but these issues currently are at the forefront for clinicians faced with the need for evidence-based practice decisions involving children with highly unintelligible speech. It is important to remember, however, that as we make progress in answering one question, additional questions often will arise.

APPENDIXES

Consonant Classifications Chart

	/p/	/b/	/t/	/d/	/k/	/g/	/f/	/v/	/θ/	/ð/	/s/	/z/	/ʃ/	/ʒ/	/tʃ/	/dʒ/	/m/	/n/	/ŋ/	/r/	/l/	/w/	/j/	/h/
Obstruents	X	X	X	X	X	X	X	X	X	X	X	X	X	X	X	X								X
Sonorants																	X	X	X	X	X	X	X	
Stops	X	X	X	X	X	X																		
Fricatives							X	X	X	X	X	X	X	X										X
Affricates															X	X								
Liquids																				X	X			
Nasals																	X	X	X					
Glides																						X	X	
Stridents							X	X			X	X	X	X	X	X								
Sibilants											X	X	X	X	X	X								
Labials	X	X					X	X									X					X		
Interdentals									X	X														
Alveolars			X	X							X	X						X			X			
Palatals													X	X	X	X				X			X	
Velars					X	X													X					
Glottals																								X
Voiced		X		X		X		X		X		X		X		X	X	X	X	X	X	X	X	
Voiceless	X		X		X		X		X		X		X		X									X

From *Targeting Intelligible Speech* (2nd ed.; p. 176), by B. Hodson and E. Paden, 1991, Austin, TX: Pro-Ed. © 1991 by Barbara Williams Hodson and Elaine Pagel Paden. Adapted with permission.

Eliciting Consonants/Patterns— Some Suggestions for Children with Highly Unintelligible Speech

Some General Suggestions

There are several steps that practitioners generally follow, starting with the simplest method and then adding assists as needed until the desired production is obtained. Typically the process begins by the clinician modeling a sound (or a pattern) in a monosyllabic word first and then asking the child to imitate the production. If that does not yield the appropriate response, the next step involves modeling/imitating the sound in isolation.

Two additional assists are added as needed: tactile and visual cues. For example, the clinician often says, "Watch my mouth," while modeling and then may touch where the sound is to be produced (general location outside mouth or specific place inside the mouth). If none of these steps succeed, slight amplification is added with the clinician holding the microphone near his or her mouth while modeling and then placing the microphone near the child's mouth while he or she imitates.

It is imperative, of course, that clinicians be thoroughly familiar with basic phonetics, particularly place, manner, and voicing characteristics of consonants. This knowledge will provide the foundation for eliciting most consonants. There are, however, some consonants/patterns that commonly require special efforts. Specific suggestions for additional assists are provided in the following sections.

Consonants/Patterns That Often Are Difficult for Children with Expressive Phonological Impairment

Velar Stops

Children with highly unintelligible speech typically substitute an alveolar /t, d/ or the glottal stop /ʔ/ for velars /k, g/, or they may omit velars in certain word positions (e.g., final consonants). A technique that has served as an additional assist for children who do not succeed with the common assists mentioned in the preceding paragraphs has been to model and have the child imitate the velar fricative /x/. This seems to disrupt their matching an alveolar (or glottal stop) for a velar and helps them develop an accurate kinesthetic image involving the velar place of articulation. After the child has developed the ability to produce a velar fricative, the production can then be shaped for a velar stop. (REMINDER: /k/ should be targeted in word-final position before word-initial position.)

Sibilants

/s/ Clusters

The most common deviations for /s/ are omissions in consonant clusters and substitution of a stop at the same place of articulation (i.e., /t/). It has been found that it is more expedient for children with highly unintelligible speech to target /s/ clusters before /s/ singleton because when prevocalic singleton /s/ is stimulated first, the child typically retains the substituted stop (e.g., [stoʊp] for *soap).* Word-initial /s/ clusters (e.g., /sp, st, sm, sn/) are usually facilitated first. A tactile cue that has been an effective assist has been to draw a finger up the child's arm while producing /s/ and then to tap the arm for the second consonant production. For word-final /s/ clusters (e.g., /ts, ps/), a different cue (e.g., rapid pointing toward child's mouth) is used to reduce the child's initial tendency to produce /s/ at the beginning (e.g., [sboʊ] instead of *boats).* By approximately the third cycle, word-initial /s/ clusters are embedded in "It's a _____" phrases (e.g., *It's a spoon).* After a child demonstrates emergence/generalization of /s/ clusters in spontaneous utterances, it may be necessary to spend a few hours on word-medial and word-final internal /s/ clusters (e.g., *basket, desk).* In addition, some children need to spend an hour on singleton /s/ if an intrusive stop is still occurring. The technique that helps children in this situation is to model a short /s/ and to exaggerate and prolong the vowel that follows (e.g., [si:]). (REMINDER: It is imperative to model a soft precise /s/.)

Palatals /s, ʒ, ʧ, ʤ/

Depalatalization (e.g., [su] for *shoe)* is fairly common. A technique that has served to facilitate productions of palatal sibilants has been to incorporate the palatal glide /j/ in models (e.g., [sj] for /ʃ/; i.e., [sju] for *shoe).* This helps the child develop an accurate kinesthetic image. Coalesence occurs soon after (along the lines of adult productions of [mɪʃu] for *miss you).* Models for the other palatal sibilants are [zj] for /ʒ/; [ʧj] for /ʧ/; and [ʤj] for /ʤ/.

Liquids

Prevocalic /l/

The most common substitution for prevocalic /l/ is /w/; the second most common is /j/. A practice that has been effective for most children has been to teach them to click the tongue tip against the alveolar ridge with the mouth open slightly. The child needs to do this clicking by raising the tongue tip (not the mandible). After children learn to do this, they are encouraged to practice tongue-tip clicking every day for a week. At the beginning of the following session, the child sometimes produces a tongue-tip click then names the prevocalic /l/ word. The clicking is faded as the child gains facility producing /l/.

Prevocalic /r/

The glide /w/ is by far the most common substitution for /r/. Productions of /r/ are stimulated for approximately an hour at the end of each cycle. The initial step is to teach the child to produce carefully selected production-practice words without inserting/substituting /w/. The first step involves the clinician modeling /ɝ/ and then exaggerating the following vowel. During beginning cycles, the production/ʊ/ is accepted initially but /w/ would not be acceptable. The child is also taught to open his or her mouth wide, not allowing lip rounding. This task is extremely difficult for children at first, but it lays a beginning foundation. By the second or third cycle (after the child demonstrates successful productions of velars), /kr, gr/ words are targeted because velars tend to facilitate productions of /r/. This method has been found to help children (especially preschoolers) progress gradually toward adequate productions of /r/.

Sample Motivational/Experiential-Play Production-Practice Activities

- **Flashlight Game** (hiding cards or objects; then finding them with a flashlight)
- **Fishing** (with magnet and paper clips)
- **Basketball, Baseball, Volleyball, Bowling, Golf**
- **Mailbox** (naming, then mailing cards)
- **Theater** (e.g., acting out /s/ cluster words)
- **Themes** (e.g., camping)
- **Children's Board Games**
- **Feed the Clown or an Animal**
- **Pin the ____ on the _____**
- **What's Missing?**
- **Taking Photos with a Camera** (toy or digital)
- **Finding Items for a Day's Target** (e.g., *rock)*
- **Finding Buried Objects** (in a box of sand or styrofoam pellets)
- **Taking Cards or Objects from Pockets**
- **Roll or Pitch a Ball or Beanbag** (landing on or knocking over cards)
- **Binoculars** (looking for cards or objects)
- **Making a Road with Cards** (then driving a vehicle, stopping, and then naming)
- **Household Activities** (e.g., cooking)
- **Making Spoon & Sponge Collages**
- **Tic-Tac-Toe or Stic-Stac-Stoe**
- **Matching/Concentration/What's Missing?**
- **Variations of Hopping on** (and naming) **Cards**
- **Building Activities** (blocks, Legos®)
- **Shopping**
- **Musical Chairs**
- **Puppets**
- **Puzzles**
- **Craft Activities**

Objects and large cards (5" x 8") are used as stimuli to elicit naming responses. The child must say the target pattern appropriately (e.g., /sp/ in *spoon)* and then "take a turn" (e.g., throw the basketball into the hoop). Then the next card or object is named, and the child gets to take a turn again. Typically clinicians spend 8 to 10 minutes on an activity.

Major Phonological Assessment Tools: Tests & Software

Test	Description	Age Range	Author(s)	Publisher
Assessment Link between Phonology and Articulation (ALPHA–R)	50 black & white drawings; sentence imitation	3:00 to 8:11	Lowe, 1995	ALPHA Speech and Language Resources
Bankson-Bernthal Test of Phonology (BBTOP)	Assesses whole-word accuracy, traditional consonant articulation, & phonological processes	3:0 to 9:0	Bankson & Bernthal, 1990	Special Press
Clinical Assessment of Articulation and Phonology® (CAAP®)	Provides articulation inventory & provides Phonological Process Checklists	2:6-8:11	Secord & Donahue, 2002	Super Duper® Publications
Diagnostic Evaluation of Articulation and Phonology (DEAP)	Assesses articulation, phonology, & oral motor	3:0-6:11	Dodd, Hua, Crosbie, Holm, & Ozanne, 2003	Psychological Corporation®
Hodson Assessment of Phonological Patterns (HAPP–3)	Uses objects & pictures to elicit 50 stimulus words; results used for identifying major phonological patterns needing intervention	2 to any age if intelligibility is an issue (norms for 3:0 to 8:0)	Hodson, 2004	Pro-Ed
Khan-Lewis Phonological Analysis (KLPA–2)	Provides a phonological analysis using pictures from the Goldman-Fristoe Test of Articulation	2 to 21	Khan & Lewis, 2002	American Guidance Service
Smit-Hand Articulation and Phonology Evaluation (SHAPE)	80 color photos	3:0-9:0	Smit & Hand, 1997	Western Psychological Services®

Software	*Description*	*Author(s)*	*Publisher*
Computerized Articulation and Phonology Evaluation Systems (CAPES)	Analyzes articulation and phonology	Masterson & Bernhardt, 2001	Psychological Corporation®
Computerized Profiling (Version 9.7.0)	Performs phonological analysis & measures of PCC, syllable structure, PMLU, & PWP	Long, Fey, & Channell, 2006	Marquette University
Hodson Computerized Analysis of Phonological Patterns (HCAPP)	Analyzes children's phonological systems based on phonetic transcriptions of 50 words	Hodson, 2003	Phonocomp Software
LIPP: Logical International Phonetics Programs (Version 2.10)	Performs phonetic transcription on speech samples	Intelligent Hearing Systems, 2001	Intelligent Hearing Systems
PEPPER: Programs to Examine Phonetic and Phonologic Evaluation Records	A series of speech analysis programs designed to examine phonetic, phonologic, and prosodic aspects of normal and disordered speech	Shriberg, Allen, McSweeny, & Wilson, 2001	University of Wisconsin-Madison

Phonological Awareness Assessment Tools

Test	*Description*	*Author(s)*	*Publisher*
Comprehensive Test of Phonological Processing (CTOPP)	Designed for individuals from 5:0 to 24:11 years; divided into two versions; core subtests intended for 5- & 6-year-old children; consists of measures of word & phoneme deletion skills (elision tasks), syllable & phoneme blending skills, & **phoneme identity** (sound matching tasks); subtests tapping other phonological processing skills are rapid color naming, rapid object naming, digit memory, & nonword repetition tasks	Wagner, Torgesen, & Rashotte, 1999	Pro-Ed
Dynamic Indicators of Basic Early Literacy Skills (DIBELS)	Provides a set of measures that are designed to monitor early literacy development, including phonological awareness development in children kindergarten to grade 3; series of one-minute assessment probes are administered at regular intervals during the school year (e.g., beginning, middle, & end)	Good & Kaminski, 2002	Institute for the Development of Educational Achievement
Lindamood Auditory Conceptualization Test (LAC–3)	Identification & manipulation of phonemes for ages 5 years to 18-11	Lindamood & Lindamood, 2004	Pro-Ed
Phonological Abilities Test (PAT)	Normative data for children ages 4:0 to 7:11; measures skills in rhyme detection, rhyme production, word completion (syllable & phoneme), phoneme **deletion**, speech rate, & letter knowledge	Muter, Hulme, & Snowling, 1997	Psychological Corporation®

Test	Description	Author(s)	Publisher
Phonological Awareness Literacy Screening for Preschool (PALS–PreK)	Phonological awareness screening measure (designed for 4-year-old children), measures both rhyme awareness & early phoneme awareness (Other screening tests in this series include PALS–K for children in kindergarten & PALS 1–3 for children in grades 1–3)	Invernizzi, Sullivan, & Meier, 2002 Invernizzi, Meier, & Juel, 2002 Invernizzi, Meier, Swank, & Juel, 2002	University of Virginia Press
Phonological Awareness Skills Program Test (PASP)	Designed for children from 4 to 11 years; deletion skills at the word, syllable, & phoneme levels; second section focuses on phoneme manipulation skills	Rosner, 1999	Pro-Ed
The Phonological Awareness Test (PAT)	Designed for children from 5 to 9 years; measures a range of rhyming, segmentation, isolation, deletion, substitution, & blending skills; evaluates children's letter knowledge, word decoding, & invented spelling skills	Robertson & Salter, 1997	LinguiSystems
Preschool and Primary Inventory of Phonological Awareness (PIPA)	Designed for children ages 3:0 to 6:11; measures skills at the syllable, onset-rime, & phoneme level, as well as letter-sound knowledge	Dodd, Crosbie, MacIntosh, Teitzel, & Ozanne, 2000	Psychological Corporation®
Test of Phonological Awareness (TOPA)	Measures the ability of 5- to 8-year-old children to isolate phonemes in spoken words	Torgesen & Bryant, 1994	Pro-Ed
Test of Phonological Awareness Skills (TOPAS)	Designed for 5- to 10-year-old children; consists of four subtests to evaluate rhyming knowledge, ability to complete multisyllabic words, phoneme sequencing, & phoneme deletion ability	Newcomer & Barenbaum, 2003	Pro-Ed

Major Phonological Awareness Resources: Intervention Programs

Product	*Author(s)*	*Publisher*
The Gillon Phonological Awareness Training Programme	Gillon, 2000	University of Canterbury
Go-To Guide for Phonological Awareness	Sterling-Orth, 2004	Super Duper® Publications
Ladders to Literacy	Notari-Syverson, O'Connor, & Vadasy, 1998	Brookes
The Lindamood Phoneme Sequencing Program for Reading, Spelling, and Speech	Lindamood & Lindamood, 1998	Pro-Ed
The Literacy Link	Northrup, 2002	Super Duper® Publications
Once Upon a Sound	Smith-Kiewel & Molenaar Claeys, 1998	Super Duper® Publications
Phonological Awareness Skills Program	Rosner, 1999	Pro-Ed
Phonological Awareness Success	Walsh, 2002	Super Duper® Publications
Phonemic Awareness in Young Children: A Classroom Curriculum	Adams, Foorman, Lundberg, & Beeler, 1997	Brookes
Road to the Code: A Phonological Awareness Program for Young Children	Blachman, Ball, Black, & Tangel, 2000	Brookes
SillySongs	Banker, 1998	Super Duper® Publications

Product	Author(s)	Publisher
Silly Sounds Playground: Building Children's Phonological Awareness	McKinley, Schreiber, Sterling-Orth, & Tobalsky, 1999	Super Duper® Publications
Sound Linkage: An Integrated Programme for Overcoming Reading Difficulties	Hatcher, 1994	Whurr
Sounds Abound: Listening, Rhyming and Reading	Catts & Vartianen, 1993	LinguiSystems
A Sound Way: Phonological Awareness Activities for Early Literacy	Love & Reilly, 1995	Longman
Sourcebook of Phonological Awareness Activities: Children's Classic Literature	Goldsworthy, 1998	Singular/ Thomson Learning
Working Out with Phonological Awareness	Schreiber, Sterling-Orth, Thurs, & McKinley, 2000	Super Duper® Publications

Glossary

Accountability. Responsibility for diagnostic and treatment decisions.

Acoustic phonetics. A branch of phonetics dealing with the study of speech properties, including frequency, intensity, and duration.

Affricates. Consonants that begin as a stop and are released as a fricative (/ʧ/ and /ʤ/).

Affrication. Changing a nonaffricate (e.g., fricative) consonant target to an affricate (e.g., /ʃ/→/ʧ/).

Age of customary production. Age at which 51% of children produced a sound correctly in at least two positions.

Ages of suppression. The ages at which various phonological processes/deviations no longer apply for children with typical phonological acquisition.

Allophones. Variants of a phoneme in a particular language; allophones of a phoneme are generally very similar to one another (e.g., aspirated /p/ and unaspirated /p/ in English).

Alphabetic knowledge. Knowledge of the letters of the alphabet, including knowing the names of the letters and the common speech sounds to which the letters correspond.

Alveolars. Consonants produced at the alveolar ridge behind upper teeth (e.g., /l/).

Anterior consonants. Consonants produced in the front part of the oral/nasal cavities (i.e., alveolars, labials, interdentals).

Anterior/Posterior contrasts. Using posterior (e.g., velars) and anterior (e.g., alveolars) contrastively (e.g., *tea* vs. *key).*

Apraxia/Dyspraxia. Motor programming difficulty, particularly involving consonant sequences; diagnostic label currently preferred by the American Speech-Language-Hearing Association for children is "suspected Childhood Apraxia of Speech (sCAS)."

Articulation. Movements of the speech production mechanism (e.g., tongue) to produce speech sounds.

Articulation hierarchy. Progression of steps in intervention from no articulatory context (isolated phoneme production) to conversational speaking.

Articulatory Phoneticians. Those who use procedures for analyzing airflow, muscle potentials, and the movement of structures such as the tongue, lips, or jaw.

Assimilation. A sound change in which one sound is influenced by another and changes to become more similar (or identical) to it; in progressive assimilation the sound changed follows the one that has influenced it (e.g., *spoon*→[spum]; in regressive assimilation the sound changed precedes the one that influenced it (e.g., *spoon*→[fpum]).

Auditory awareness. Ability to accurately perceive sound.

Auditory discrimination. The ability to recognize a difference between two productions by a speaker.

Auditory stimulation/input. Auditorily providing productions of words containing the target pattern to enhance the individual's auditory awareness of phonological patterns.

Autism Theory. A theory of speech sound acquisition based on talking birds that emphasizes the emotional relationship between the "caregiver" and the "learner," as well as the role of selective reinforcement.

Back vowels. Production involving elevation of the back of the tongue from its neutral or rest position.

Backing. Substitution of a posterior consonant (i.e., /k/, /g/, /ŋ/, /h/) for an anterior target.

Baseline. Level of production before the onset of intervention.

Bilabial. Consonants produced by both lips (e.g., /b/).

Binary. Having two values (+ and –), as in Distinctive Feature Theory.

Carryover. Using target sounds/patterns in other word positions, other words, and other situations; a primary intervention goal.

Central vowels. Vowels produced with the middle of the tongue elevated or in its neutral or rest position.

Child phonology. The study of children's typically developing phonological systems.

Clinical phonology. Application of phonological theories and concepts to clinical problems in assessment and intervention (dating back to about 1970).

Cluster creation. Change in the output from a singleton consonant to a cluster (e.g., *see*→[sti]).

Coalescence. Replacement of two adjacent sounds by one new consonant that retains features of both original consonants (e.g., /sm/→[f]).

Coarticulation. The related, overlapping articulatory influences that occur as sounds are produced in connected speech.

Coda. Word/syllable ending.

Cognates. Consonant sounds that differ from each other only by voicing; place and manner of articulation are the same (e.g., /p/ and /b/).

Cognitive Theory. A phonological acquisition theory that stresses the creativity of the child and purports that children invent their own phonological rules by "active experimentation" and the use of strategies; also referred to as Interactionist-Discovery Theory.

COMPLEX/NOT COMPLEX. An Optimality Theory constraint specifying which sequences of consonants in a syllable are prohibited.

COMPLEX PHONEME AWARENESS TASKS. Tasks that require demonstration of multiple phonological awareness skills (e.g., both phoneme segmentation and phoneme blending) to complete them successfully.

COMPLEX SUBSTITUTIONS. Substitutions of one phoneme for another in which the error sound differs from the target sound by more than one feature (e.g., /s/→[d], involving both stopping and voicing).

CONCOMITANT. Coexisting conditions that contribute to communication difficulties.

CONFRONTATION ACTIVITIES. Learning through "conflict and reflection."

CONSONANT. A sound that is produced by a partially or completely constricted vocal tract.

CONSONANT CLUSTER. Two or more contiguous consonants in the same syllable (e.g., ***tr****ee*).

CONSONANT SEQUENCE/CLUSTER DELETION. Deletion of consonants in a sequence in the output (e.g., *street*→[it]).

CONSONANT SEQUENCE/CLUSTER REDUCTION. Omission of consonants in a sequence in the output (e.g., *tree*→[ti]).

CONSONANT SEQUENCES. Two or more contiguous consonants, including those that cross syllable and word boundaries (e.g., *ba**sk**et*).

CONSONANT SINGLETONS. Consonants surrounded by vowels or silence (i.e., no contiguous consonant).

CONSTITUENT PROCESSES/DEVIATIONS. Complex substitutions involving more than one deviation (e.g., /s/→[d]; both stopping and voicing).

CONSTRAINT TABLE/TABLEAU. In Optimality Theory, a table that shows possible productions of a word or a set of similar words, along with the relevant constraints.

CONTEXT FREE. A sound change that takes place across contexts and environments (i.e., the sound change is not limited to a particular context).

CONTEXT SENSITIVE. A sound change that takes place only in specific phonetic contexts or environments.

CONTEXTUAL FACILITATION. Selecting production practice words with optimal phonetic environment, considering adjacent sounds, position in word/syllable, and syllable stress; progression from facilitative phonetic environment to less facilitative phonetic environment.

Continuants. Produced with a continuing airflow; one of the two binary feature nodes dominated by the root node in Feature Geometry.

Continuous conversational speech sample. Spontaneous conversation or story retelling (in contrast to single-word naming).

Continuum. Continuous levels (vs. discrete).

Coronal. Produced with the blade of the tongue (e.g., alveolars); in Feature Geometry, one of the "articulator nodes."

Criterion. An expected standard or level of accuracy required.

Critical Age Hypothesis. The premise that children are at risk for literacy problems if severe speech difficulties have not resolved by age 5:6.

Cycle. Time period (typically 2 to 3 months) during which phonological patterns (typically three to six) are targeted in succession for at least 2 hours each; patterns are recycled until they emerge in spontaneous speech.

Deaffrication. Loss of either the stop or fricative component of an affricate (e.g., /ʧ/→/t/ or /ʃ/).

Decoding. Reading a printed word through relating the letters in the word to corresponding speech sounds.

Delayed imitation. A speech act when an individual does not name an item spontaneously and the examiner provides the name and then says several other words before asking the individual to say the name (contrasted with direct/immediate imitation).

Deletion rule. Phonological rule pertaining to the omission of a sound, class of sounds, or sequence of sounds.

Dental. A consonant sound produced with contact of the tongue and teeth.

Depalatalization. Substitution of a nonpalatal consonant for a palatal one (e.g., /ʃ/→/s/).

Descriptive linguistics. An approach to the study of language followed in the first part of the 20th century, which focused on determining the phonemes used in a language (also known as American Structuralism).

Diacritics (markings). Special marks used with the symbols of the International Phonetic Alphabet to add more detail to phonetic transcription (e.g., for distortions).

Diadochokinetic rate. Length of time required or number of productions for tasks (e.g., rapid repetitions of /pʌtʌkʌ/).

Diagnostic evaluation. In-depth assessment to determine if a communication disorder exists, whether intervention is needed, and the severity level of involvement (contrasted with screening).

Dialect. A variety of a language spoken by a group.

Digraph. Two letters yielding one sound (e.g., *sh).*

Diminutive. Addition of /i/ (in English) to a word; frequently observed in speech of 2-year-olds with typical development (e.g., *sheepie).*

Diphthong. Two vowels produced consecutively in the same syllable by moving the articulators smoothly from the position of one to the other so that together they serve as the nucleus of the syllable (e.g., /aɪ/).

Discontinuity. The view held by Jakobson that prelinguistic vocalizations (such as babbling) are not related to meaningful speech.

Disorder/Impairment. A condition in which productions differ to an extent that there is an interference in communication.

Disordered phonological system. Overall deviations independent of etiological factors, including childhood apraxia of speech as well as phonological disorders.

Distinctive features. A universal set of phonetic characteristics that differentiate speech sounds (e.g., [+] voice; [–] nasal). Each phoneme differs from all other phonemes by at least one distinctive feature.

Distinctive Feature Theory. Premise that phonemes are made up of distinctive phonetic properties/universal features.

Distortion. Deviation in production that is nonphonemic (e.g., lisp).

Dorsal. A sound produced with the back of the tongue (e.g., velars); one of the "articulator nodes" in Feature Geometry.

Early developing patterns/phonemes. Patterns/phonemes that typically are produced earliest by young children (e.g., CV, stops).

Ease of perception. Phonological acquisition theory which holds that easily discriminable sounds are learned first.

Elicitation. Prompting/cuing a response for a sound/word production.

Epenthesis. A type of sound change in which a sound is added within a word (e.g., *blue*→[bəlu]).

Establishment. Phase one of intervention when correct production of phonemes in isolation is the goal.

Etiological factors. Factors that may have a causal relationship to the disorder (e.g., predisposing, perpetuating).

Evidence-based practices. Approaches in which current, high-quality research evidence is considered in clinical decision making.

Experiential-play. Production-practice activities that are motivational for a child resulting in their enjoying practice of the target pattern in words.

Expressive phonological impairment. Speech sound disorder characterized by phonologically based (rather than phonetic/motoric based) speech errors.

Facilitative phonetic environment. Word structures that increase the potential for accurate production of target sound.

Feature changing rule. A phonological rule that changes a feature (e.g., voicing) contrasted with a rule that adds or deletes an entire segment.

Feature Geometry. A nonlinear theory that focuses on the features that comprise segments; features are organized in hierarchies, with some features "dominating" others.

Feature Spreading. When a quality of one sound transfers or assimilates to another.

First-word stage. Period when the first meaningful word is produced.

Foot. A metrical unit consisting of a strong (stressed) syllable and one or two weak syllables.

Fricatives. Consonants produced with partial blockage of the breath stream causing turbulence or friction during production.

Front vowels. Vowels that are produced with a forward shift of the tongue from its neutral or rest position.

Frontal/interdental lisp. Tongue protrusion during production of sibilants with stridency maintained (not a substitution of /θ/).

Fronting. Replacement of a posterior consonant by an anterior consonant (e.g., /k/→[θ]).

Functional tiers. In Gestural/Articulatory Phonology, the tiers that allow for overlap between consonants and vowels.

Generalization. Successful transfer of learned sounds to related unlearned sounds.

Generative Phonology. Phonological theory that includes formal phonological rules and abstract underlying rules to describe the sound system of a language.

Gestural Phonology. Phonological theory in which the phonological system is based on articulation; also referred to as Articulatory Phonology.

Gestural score. In Gestural Phonology, a gestural score represents, on different levels of tiers, several movements (or gestures) that may overlap in time.

Gesture (Articulatory). A basic unit of Gestural Phonology; an abstract characterization of an articulatory event.

Glides. Prevocalic consonants characterized by a rapid movement of the articulations from a high front or high back tongue arch to the vowel that follows; /w/ and /j/.

Gliding. Replacement of a nonglide consonant with a glide (e.g., /l/→/j/).

Glottal. Consonant produced by completely or partially constricting the glottis (space between the vocal folds).

Glottal stop replacement. Substitution of a glottal stop for a consonant.

Grapheme. Written or printed letters; may or may not correspond to phonemes.

Hierarchical relationships. Relationships among linguistic units, such as syllables and segments, on different levels or tiers, with each tier being dominated by the tier above; a basic concept in Nonlinear Phonology.

High-amplitude sucking technique. Research method that tests speech perception in infants from birth to 5 months of age.

High vowels. Vowels produced with the tongue raised above its neutral or rest position.

Homonym. One phonetic form representing two (or more) different words (e.g., *vase* and *plane* both realized as [be]).

Homonymy. Production of the same phonetic form for two or more words that normally are not produced the same (e.g., [ti] for both *see* and *tea).*

Iambic. A "right prominent" foot, made up of a weak syllable followed by a strong syllable (e.g., *tonight).*

Idiolect. Speech that is characteristic of a single individual.

Idiosyncratic rules. Preferred productions by a child that are unusual/unexpected.

Implicational universals. A tenet of Jakobson's Universal Order Theory that purports to account for phoneme inventories and for the order in which children acquire phonemes; for example, "back ⊃ front" means that if a language has back sounds it also will have front sounds and also predicts that children will acquire front sounds before they acquire similar back sounds.

Independent analysis. Determination of the sounds and syllable structures produced independent of adult words and meaning; contrasted with relational analysis.

Individualized education programs. Special education services, provided as a federal mandate for "free and appropriate public education" in order to address the needs of students with eligible handicapping conditions.

Input/Output. Input is whatever is immediately to the left and output is whatever is immediately to the right of the arrow in a phonological rule.

Integrative rehearsal. Production-practice to enhance auditory and kinesthetic feedback and self-monitoring.

Intelligibility. The degree to which others can understand a person's speech; speech that is "highly unintelligible" is extremely difficult for listeners to understand.

Interacting. Two or more phonological processes/deviations that apply to a particular sound or cluster, giving rise to a complex substitution (e.g., initial voicing interacting with velar fronting, resulting in a substitution of [d] for /k/).

Interactionist-Discovery theory. See **Cognitive Theory**.

Interdentals. Consonants produced with the tongue usually touching the upper and lower teeth so that a fricative airflow is produced.

International Phonetic Alphabet. Symbols that have been assigned for each phoneme across all of the world's languages (originally developed in 1886, last revised in 2005).

International Phonetic Association. Organization of phoneticians promoting the study of phonetics as a science.

Intervocalic. Sequential position of consonant(s) between two vowels.

Kinesthetic. The sense/awareness of positions or movements of articulatory structures.

Knowledge types. A continuum of six categories developed by Elbert and Gierut to rank children's "productive phonological knowledge" from the most knowledge (type 1) to the least (type 6).

Labials. Sounds produced with the lips (bilabials and labiodentals); one of the "articulator nodes" in Feature Geometry.

Labiodental. A consonant that is produced by the lower lip contacting the upper-front teeth.

Laryngeal. Produced at the larynx; the laryngeal node in Feature Geometry dominates features that concern voicing.

Lateral lisp. Distortion involving sibilants where airstream is directed laterally; stridency is maintained.

Letter-name knowledge. The ability to name letters of the alphabet and to specify their corresponding sounds.

Lexical acquisition. The acquisition of vocabulary words or "lexical items," said to be closely tied to phonological acquisition at the earliest stages.

Limitation. One of the mechanisms by which the innate phonological system is revised, according to Stampe; as the child progresses, natural phonological processes may apply in fewer environments or to fewer sound classes.

Linear Theories. Theories, such as Generative Phonology and Natural Phonology, that focus mainly on strings of segments (consonants and vowels) on a level or tier.

Linguistic. The period of language use that occurs once a true word is spoken.

Liquids. Sounds for which the articulators make only partial, frictionless approximation (i.e., /l/ and /r/).

Literacy difficulties. Problems with written language (e.g., reading, writing, and spelling).

Low vowels. Vowels produced with the tongue lowered from its neutral or rest position.

Maintenance. Continued accuracy of sound production as measured at periodic follow-up sessions (e.g., 1 month or 6 months after intervention has ended).

Major substitutions. Replacing one sound with another.

Manner of articulation. The modification of air flowing through the oral and nasal cavities by the articulators.

Markedness. A complex phonological concept that concerns differences among sounds, with a "marked" sound having an added phonetic property, such as voicing, compared to voiceless cognate.

"Matthew Effects." Stanovich compared achievement levels of children who are poor beginning readers with their peers who have good decoding skills and noted that the gap widens over the years (rather than staying parallel); (the "rich get richer and the poor get poorer").

Mental/Lexical representations. The hypothesized "underlying representations" or forms of words stored mentally to which phonological rules apply.

Metalinguistic Skills. The ability to think and talk about word structures.

Metathesis. Transposition/reversal of sounds or sequences (e.g., *ask*→[æks].

Metrical Phonology. A nonlinear theory that focuses on syllable structure and prosodic features such as word stress and tone.

Mid vowels. Vowels produced with the tongue in a neutral position.

Migration. Movement of a sound in the output to another position in the word (e.g., *smoke*→[moks]).

Minimal contrast. A sound segment distinction by which two morphemes or words differ in pronunciation.

Minimal pair. Two words differing by only one sound (e.g., *pat* and *bat);* the test for determining the phonemes of a language.

Minimal place of articulation shifts. Changes in articulation that are near the target (e.g., /θ/→[f]); typically these do not have a particularly adverse effect on intelligibility.

Monosyllabic. Consisting of one syllable.

Morphemes. Minimal meaningful linguistic units; may involve more than one phoneme.

Morphophonemic alternations. Alternations between two or more forms of a morpheme, with accompanying variations in the sounds that make up the morpheme (e.g., *house, houses).*

Multisyllabic. Containing more than one syllable.

Multisyllabicity. Ability of individuals above the age of 8 years to produce complex multisyllabic words (e.g., *extraneous).*

Nasalization. The inappropriate addition of nasal resonance to a non-nasal sound.

Nasals. Consonants produced by blocking the oral cavity and emitting the sound through the nasal cavity.

Natural phoneme classes. Groups of closely related sounds that share phonetic properties (e.g., stridents) that undergo the same sound changes.

Natural phonological processes. According to Natural Phonology, an innate phonological system.

Natural Phonology. A phonological acquisition theory developed by Stampe in which natural processes are the central concept.

Natural process analysis. Analyzing phonetically motivated sound changes (e.g., cluster reduction) that occur in typically developing children across languages; excludes deviations such as backing and initial consonant deletion.

Neutral vowels. Vowels produced with the tongue in its rest position, typical of the position for the schwa.

Neutralization. Merging of a phonemic contrast of a language, generally in a particular position or context. For example, the contrast between /t/ and /d/ is neutralized between stressed and unstressed vowels in English, where both phonemes are replaced by a flap.

Nonlinear Theories. Theories, such as Feature Geometry and Metrical Phonology (sometimes referred to as "multilinear"), that focus on linguistic units, such as syllables and segments that occur on different levels or tiers, in contrast to "linear" theories.

Not complex (Onset). Also written as *Complex (Onset); a constraint from Optimality Theory, which states that onsets cannot be complex; that is, a syllable cannot begin with a consonant cluster (a complex onset).

Nucleus. The sonority peak or loudest part of a syllable, usually a vowel, although sometimes a syllabic consonant.

Obstruents. Consonants made with the vocal tract airflow partially or totally impeded (i.e., stops, fricatives, and affricates).

Omissions. Sound or syllable deletions.

Onset. One or more consonants (up to three in English) that precede the vowel/nucleus.

Onset-rime units. Syllables that can be segmented into an onset (i.e., one or more consonants that precede a vowel) and a rime unit (the vowel plus the following consonant[s]). For example, in the word *stop, st* is the onset and *op* is the rime unit.

Opposition. Contrasts among the phonemes of a language; the properties by which the phonemes of a language contrast with one another (e.g., voicing); minimal, maximal, and multiple oppositions.

Optimal match. The aspect that is slightly above an individual's current level of functioning so that the learner is challenged but successful.

Optimality Theory. A theory of phonology developed in the 1990s that focuses on constraints.

Ordering. In Natural Phonology, one of the mechanisms by which the innate phonological system is revised; as the child progresses, processes may be sequenced such that one cannot apply after (and to the output of) another.

Output constraints. In Optimality Theory, limitations on what can be produced.

Palatals. Consonants produced when the tongue contacts or approaches some portion of the hard palate.

Palatalization. The addition of a palatal feature to a nonpalatal target (e.g., /s/→[ʃ]).

Percentage of Consonants Correct. A procedure developed by Shriberg and Kwiatkowski that involves determining the number of consonants that are totally correct in a spontaneous speech sample and dividing by the total number of words.

Percentage of identifiable/intelligible words. A procedure that involves having an unfamiliar listener write the words that are intelligible in a child's speech.

Phone. A single speech sound produced by a speaker; may not be meaningful.

Phoneme. One of a group of similar speech sounds that are perceived within a language as the same; differentiates meaning in a language; phonemes vary from language to language.

Phonemic awareness. Awareness (independent of meaning) that words comprise individual speech sounds or phonemes (e.g., awareness that the word *cat* can be segmented into /k/ /æ/ /t/).

Phoneme blending. Blending individual phonemes together to form a word (e.g., blending /ʃ/ /i/ /p/ together to form the word *sheep).*

Phoneme deletion. Omitting a phoneme from a word to make a new word or nonword. (e.g., *cold* without the /k/ sound is *old).*

Phoneme identity. Identifying phonemes in words (e.g., the first sound in the word *dog* is /d/).

Phoneme-grapheme relationships. The relationship between a phoneme (individual speech sound) and its grapheme (alphabet letter or letters); (e.g., understanding the relationship between the speech sound /f/ and the letter *f* or the letters *ph).*

Phoneme manipulation. Changing or omitting phonemes in words (e.g., changing the word *cat* to *cap).*

Phoneme-oriented. Focus of assessment or intervention is on individual phonemes (contrasted with patterns).

Phoneme segmentation. Segmenting a word into its individual phonemes (e.g., segmenting the word *speak* into /s/ /p/ /i/ /k/).

Phonemics. The approach to phonology (followed by descriptive linguists) that focused on determining the phonemes and allophones used in a language.

Phonetic repertoire. All of the speech sounds that an individual produces.

Phonetic symbol. A written character that represents a particular speech segment.

Phonetics. The scientific study of speech sounds, their form, substance, and perception, and the application of this study to an understanding and improvement of linguistic expression.

Phonetic transcription. A written account of the sound segments in a spoken language sample.

Phonological acquisition. Development of the production of speech sounds and patterns (associated with a child developing speech).

Phonological awareness. Explicit awareness of the sound structure of spoken words independent of meaning; also referred to as phonological sensitivity and metaphonological awareness; includes phonemic awareness but is more encompassing (i.e., includes syllable awareness and rhyming).

Phonological awareness intervention. Structured activities that specifically target developing an individual's awareness that words are comprised of smaller speech sound units.

Phonological deficiencies. Deviations that differ from standard productions (e.g., velar deficiencies, including omissions as well as substitutions) typically associated with children who have intelligibility issues.

Phonological deviations. Speech sound changes (e.g., omissions, substitutions) that result in productions that differ from the standard.

Phonological foundation. Development of the ability to eventually produce sounds/phonological patterns of the child's language.

Phonological mean length of utterance. A procedure that assigns points to correctly produced segments of speech.

Phonological patterns. Accepted groupings of sounds within an oral language (e.g., consonant clusters, stridents); what a child needs to produce to be understood.

Phonological processing. A broad term used to describe the use of phonological information in processing spoken and written language; phonological awareness is a subset of phonological processing.

Phonological representation. Storage of speech sound information about words in long-term memory.

Phonological rule. A formal way of capturing or showing a sound change (e.g., t→d /#_ is a substitution rule that captures the fact that /t/ is replaced by [d] in word-final position).

Phonological system. An individual's use of sounds, patterns, and rules.

Phonology. Sound system of a language and the study of the sound system.

Phonotactics. Rules of a language specifying where sounds can occur (in words or syllables) and how sounds can be combined in that language.

Physiological phonetics. A major branch of phonetics that deals with speech sound production; also called articulatory phonetics.

Place of articulation. The major point of contact or near contact of the active and passive articulators in producing a speech sound.

Positive reinforcement. In Behaviorist theories (specifically Stimulus-Response Theory), something desirable, such as praise or a small token, that immediately follows a desired response and is said to increase the likelihood of that response occurring again.

Posterior consonants. Consonant sounds articulated in the back part of oral cavity (i.e., velars and glottals).

Posterior/Anterior contrasts. Awareness and production of posterior consonants (e.g., /k/) and anterior consonants (e.g., /t/) and using these contrastively.

Postvocalic. A consonant that occurs immediately after a vowel.

Postvocalic devoicing. Loss of voicing for word-final consonants (usually preceded by vowel lengthening in English (e.g., *page* → [pei: ʧ]); considered to be a "normal" sound change in English.

Prelinguistic. Vocalization prior to the first true words.

Preventive intervention. Intervention that aims to reduce or alleviate known risks for a target population (e.g., intervention to reduce or prevent reading and spelling difficulties during the school years).

Prevocalic. A consonant that occurs immediately before a vowel.

Prevocalic devoicing. Production of a voiceless consonant for a voiced one preceding a vowel (e.g., *zip*→[sɪp]).

Prevocalic voicing. Production of a voiced consonant for a voiceless one preceding a vowel (e.g., *tea*→[di]).

Principle of maximal contrast. A principle of Jakobson's Universal Order Theory which holds that the first sounds learned are those that differ from one another by several features.

Print-referencing activities. Activities used during shared-book reading to direct children's attention to print and literacy conventions (e.g., pointing to words on a page as the words are read, commenting about specific letters on a page).

Process chronology. A listing (by Grunwell, 1987) of the ages at which various common phonological processes are suppressed.

Productive phonological knowledge. Information that is said to be stored mentally for each morpheme but derived from productions rather than perception.

Prognosis. Potential for improvement; expected outcome.

Prosodic features. Aspects of speech communication like stress and tone.

Prosodic Theory. A nonsegmental theory of phonological acquisition that emphasizes the importance of input and perception.

Prosodic word. A unit in Nonlinear Phonology that contains just one primary or main stress, often equivalent to an actual word.

Prosody/Suprasegmentals. Aspects such as stress and tone that extend over more than one segment.

Protowords. Consistent sound patterns produced by young children that are semantically similar but may not be modeled after adult words; child's first meaningful vocal productions.

Psycholinguistic. Theoretical model of speech processing from which hypotheses are generated about the level of breakdown; attends to both input and output.

Readiness. Stimulable for the production of a pattern/sound.

Reassociation. A type of rule in Feature Geometry by which features of one segment become associated with another segment, as in feature coalescence (e.g., *spoon*→ [fun]) with the labial feature of the /p/ becoming associated with the supralaryngeal node of /s/, resulting in an [f] for /sp/ substitution).

Recycled. The re-presentation of patterns during successive cycles.

Redundancy rules. Sound features that can be filled in because they are predictable or inferred.

Reduplication. Production of a series of consonant-vowel syllables in which the consonant is the same in every syllable (e.g., *mamama).*

Regular words. Words that can be decoded or spelled using knowledge of how letters relate to speech sounds (phonemes) in words (e.g., *dog, jump)* contrasted with irregular words (e.g., *they, sword).*

Reinforcement schedule. A predetermined plan for frequency of reinforcement following correct production of a target phoneme.

Relational analysis. The act of comparing productions with those of adults; contrasted with independent analysis.

Relative ranking. In Optimality Theory, constraints are ordered such that the more important ones are ranked higher than those that are less important.

Reorganization. Facilitating overall productions so that the individual reorganizes his or her own phonological system.

Repairs. In Optimality Theory, phonological processes may be viewed as "repairs" that make it possible for a child to produce forms that otherwise are "unpronounceable" because they violate constraints (e.g., cluster reduction makes it possible for a child with the constraint *Complex to produce the word *blue* as [bu]).

Re-ranking. In Optimality Theory, re-ranking of constraint accounts for children's phonological acquisition; as a child progresses, output constraints are "demoted" and faithfulness constraints are "promoted" so that the child's output eventually matches the adult form.

Resonance. The amplification of certain frequency components of the vocal fold source tone by the air-filled cavities of the vocal tract.

Response. In Behaviorist Theory, specifically, the stimulus-response (S-R) paradigm, the desired behavior (pointing to a picture, saying a specific word, etc.) that is elicited by a particular stimulus.

Rhythmic tier. In Gestural Phonology, the tier for stress levels.

Rime. Nucleus or peak of the syllable (usually a vowel), along with any consonants that follow it in the coda.

Root node. In Metrical Phonology, the node that specifies the feature content of a segment.

Rounded. Sound production containing lip rounding.

Screening. Procedures that provide preliminary information that is used to determine if further in-depth testing is needed.

Scientific method. Systematic process for formulating, testing, and accepting/rejecting/modifying hypotheses.

Segment. A speech sound (consonant or vowel or diphthong).

Segmental tier. In Metrical Phonology, the tier that shows the consonants and vowels that fill each slot of a syllable.

Selective reinforcement. A tenet of Mowrer's Autism Theory, which holds that caregivers reinforce sounds that are similar to those of the adult language, causing them to be retained, while sounds that are not similar to those of the adult language are not reinforced and therefore drop out.

Self-monitoring skills. Monitoring of one's own speech for errors.

Sensory-perceptual training. Ear training.

Severity (level). The degree to which communication ability is below expectations (e.g., moderate, severe).

Sibilants. Consonants that are produced with mid-to-high frequency turbulence.

Single-word samples. Elicited, individual words usually using objects or pictures as prompts.

Skeletal tier. In Nonlinear Phonology, the tier consisting of the consonant and vowel composition of each syllable; in Gestural Phonology, the tier that shows the syllable structure of the utterance.

Speech. A mode of language expression based on sounds emitted through the mouth and nose.

Sonorants. Sounds produced with a relatively unobstructed vocal tract (i.e., vowels, diphthongs, nasals, liquids, and glides).

Speech perception. Identification of the vowels and consonants of a language, largely from auditory cues.

Speech sample. A selection of a child's speech.

Spoonerism. The transferring of the first two sounds of syllables/words (e.g., *fit, sun→sit, fun).*

Stimulability. The ability of a child to produce a sound (that was not produced spontaneously) following a model and, if necessary, with additional assists (e.g., tactile cues, amplification).

Stimulable. Sounds that can be produced after cuing (e.g, imitating a model).

Stimulate. To provide assists to help an individual learn to produce a sound/pattern.

Stimulus. In Behavioristic theories (specifically the stimulus-response paradigm), the picture, object, verbal cue, etc., that is used to elicit a desired response.

Stopping. Substitution of a stop consonant for a fricative, liquid, nasal, or glide.

Stops. Consonants produced with complete blockage of the airflow in the oral cavity.

Stridents. Fricatives and affricates characterized by considerable turbulence caused by forceful airflow striking the back of teeth; includes sibilants and /f/ and /v/.

Strong syllable. A stressed syllable.

Substitutions. Replacing one sound with another.

Successive approximations. Gradual progression in productions toward the desired target sound.

Suppression. In Natural Phonology, one of the mechanisms by which the innate phonological system is revised; as the child progresses, processes that are not part of the adult phonological system are "overcome" and no longer apply.

Surface representations. Productions that are derived from more abstract underlying forms or representations by phonological rules.

Syllabics. Sounds that serve as syllable nuclei, including vowels, diphthongs, or syllabic consonants.

Syllable awareness. Awareness that words can be segmented into syllables: for example, being aware that the word *baby* can be divided into two syllables: /bei/ and /bi/.

Syllable/word shapes/structure. The composition of a syllable. In Nonlinear/Metrical Phonology, each syllable is said to be made up of an (optional) onset and a rime.

Syllable tier. In Metrical Phonology, the syllable tier, represented by a sigma (σ), is dominated by the word or foot tier and in turn dominates the onset-rime tier; that is, each syllable contains an optional onset and a required rime, which, in turn, must contain a vowel or syllabic consonant and may contain an optional consonant (coda).

Syllableness. The ability to produce/sequence two or more syllables.

Tactile cuing. The use of touch cues to stimulate appropriate placement or manner of production (e.g., touching under the chin at the base of the tongue to stimulate a velar production).

Target pattern. Adult syllable shape, sound sequence, or consonant category that a child needs to acquire.

Target phoneme(s). One or more phonemes within a pattern used to facilitate the development of that pattern.

Tongue protrusion. An inappropriate positioning of the tongue forward in the mouth or between the teeth.

Transfer. Sound production in nontreatment settings.

Trochaic. A "left prominent" foot, made up of a strong syllable followed by a weak syllable (e.g., *basket).*

Underlying representations. Hypothesized "mental representations" of words to which phonological rules apply; also called lexical representations or forms.

Universal. Being found in all (or nearly all) of the languages that have been studied.

Universal grammar. The part of grammar that is innate and found in all languages.

Universal Order Theory. The theory of phonological acquisition proposed by Jakobson which purports that phonemic distinctions are acquired in the same order across all the languages of the world; Laws of Irreversible Solidarity.

Valid. When an assessment produces intended results/information.

Velars. Consonants made with tongue contact on or near the soft palate (velum).

Velopharyngeal port. Those structures (soft palate, uvula, and pharyngeal wall) that open and close the connection between the oral and nasal cavities.

Velum. Soft palate.

Violations. Productions/Forms that do not obey the constraints of a language or a speaker in Optimality theory.

Virgules. A pair of backslash marks (/ /) used to denote a distinctive speech sound.

Visually reinforced head-turn method. Research procedure that tests speech perception in infants 6 to 12 months of age.

Vocables. Vocalizations that have some phonetic consistency but do not have stable sounds or meaning.

Vocalizations. Infant's early vocalizations (prelinguistic) that do not appear to be based on the adult language or to be used in a meaningful way.

Voiced. A type of sound produced with vibration of the adducted vocal folds in the larynx.

Voiceless. A type of consonant produced without vibration of the adducted vocal folds.

Vowel neutralization. Lack of a differentiation between vowels; several are reduced to the same perceived sound.

Vowelization. Replacement of a consonant (usually a postvocalic or syllabic liquid) with a vowel (referred to as vocalization by some phonologists).

Vowels. Speech sounds produced with an unobstructed vocal tract.

Weak syllable. An unstressed syllable.

Whole word accuracy. Determination of the total number of words that are produced with complete accuracy in a speech sample.

Word recognition. The ability to recognize a printed word.

Word tier. The top tier of a Metrical Phonology "tree," showing the composition of the word; the word tier dominates the foot tier, which, in turn, dominates the syllable tier.

Zone of proximal development. What the child independently and currently can do versus what potentially could be done with adequate support.

References

Adams, M. J., Foorman, B. R., Lundberg, I., & Beeler, C. (1997). *Phonemic awareness in young children: A classroom curriculum.* Baltimore: Brookes.

Adams, M. (1990). *Beginning to read: Thinking and learning about print.* Cambridge, MA: MIT Press.

Almost, D., & Rosenbaum, P. (1998). Effectiveness of speech intervention for phonological disorders: A randomized controlled trial. *Developmental Medicine & Child Neurology, 40,* 319–325.

American Speech-Language-Hearing Association (ASHA). (2001). Roles and responsibilities of speech-language pathologists with respect to reading and writing in children and adolescents (Position statement, executive summary of guidelines, technical report). *ASHA Supplement 21,* 17–27.

Anthony, J., & Lonigan, C. (2004). The nature of phonological awareness: Converging evidence from four studies of preschool and early grade school children. *Journal of Educational Psychology, 96,* 43–55.

Arlt, P. B., & Goodban, M. T. (1976). A comparative study of articulation acquisition as based on a study of 240 normals, aged three to six. *Language, Speech, and Hearing Services in Schools,* 7, 173–180.

Banker, B. (1998). *SillySongs.* Greenville, SC: Super Duper® Publications.

Bankson, N., & Bernthal, J. (1990). *Bankson-Bernthal Test of Phonology (BBTOP).* Austin, TX: Pro-Ed.

Barlow, J. A. (2001). Case study: Optimality theory and the assessment and treatment of phonological disorders. *Language, Speech, and Hearing Services in Schools, 32,* 242–256.

Barlow, J. A. (2002). Recent advances in phonological theory and treatment: Part II. *Language, Speech, and Hearing Services in Schools, 33,* 4–8.

Barlow, J. A., & Gierut, J. A. (1999). Optimality theory in phonological acquisition. *Journal of Speech and Hearing Research, 42,* 1482–1498.

Berko, J., & Brown, R. (1960). Psycholinguistic research methods. In P. Mussen (Ed.), *Handbook of research methods in child development* (pp. 517–557). New York: Wiley.

Berman, S. (2001, November). *Speech intelligibility and the Down syndrome child.* Poster session presented at the annual convention of the American Speech-Language-Hearing Association, New Orleans, LA.

Bernhardt, B. H., & Gilbert, J. G. (1992). Applying linguistic theory to speech-language pathology: The case for non-linear phonology. *Clinical Linguistics and Phonetics, 6,* 259–281.

Bernhardt, B., & Stemberger, J. (2000). *Workbook in nonlinear phonology for clinical application.* Austin, TX: Pro-Ed.

Bernhardt, B. H., & Stoel-Gammon, C. (1994). Nonlinear phonology: Introduction and clinical application. *Journal of Speech and Hearing Research, 37,* 123–143.

Bernthal, J. E., & Bankson, N. W. (Eds.). (2004). *Articulation and phonological disorders* (5th ed.). Needham Heights, MA: Allyn & Bacon.

Bird, J., Bishop, D., & Freeman, N. (1995). Phonological awareness and literacy development in children with expressive phonological impairments. *Journal of Speech and Hearing Research, 38,* 446–462.

Bishop, D., & Adams, C. (1990). A prospective study of the relationship between specific language impairment, phonological disorders, and reading retardation. *Journal of Child Psychology and Psychiatry, 31,* 1027–1050.

Blache, S. (1978). *The acquisition of distinctive features.* Baltimore: University Park Press.

Blachman, B. (1984). Relationship of rapid naming ability and language analysis skill to kindergarten and first-grade reading achievement. *Journal of Educational Psychology, 76,* 610–622.

Blachman, B., Ball, E., Black, R., & Tangel, D. (1994). Kindergarten teachers develop phoneme awareness in low-income, inner-city classrooms. *Reading and Writing: An Interdisciplinary Journal, 6*(1) 1–18.

Blachman, B., Ball, E., Black, R., & Tangel, D. (2000). *Road to the code: A phonological awareness program for young children.* Baltimore: Brookes.

Bleile, K. (2002). Evaluating articulation and phonological disorders when the clock is running. *American Journal of Speech-Language Pathology, 11,* 243–249.

Bleile, K. (2004). *Manual of articulation and phonological disorder: Infancy through adulthood* (2nd ed.). Clifton Park, NY: Thomson/Delmar Learning.

Bloomfield, L. (1933). *Language.* New York: Holt, Rinehart, & Winston.

Bosley, E. C. (1981). *Techniques for articulatory disorders.* Springfield, IL: Charles C. Thomas.

Bowey, J. (1986). Syntactic awareness in relation to reading skill and on-going reading comprehension monitoring. *Journal of Experimental Child Psychology, 41,* 282–299.

Bradley, D. P. (1989). A systematic multiple-phoneme approach. In N. Creaghead, P. Newman, & W. Secord (Eds.), *Assessment and remediation of articulatory and phonological disorders* (2nd ed.; pp. 303–322). Columbus, OH: Merrill.

Bradley, D. P., Allen, G. D., & Clifford, V. V. (1983). Reliability of assessment of articulation skills in conversational speech. *Division of Council on Communication Disorders Bulletin, 11,* 28–31.

Bradley, L., & Bryant, P. (1983). Categorizing sounds and learning to read—A causal connection. *Nature, 301,* 419–421.

Browman, C., & Goldstein, L. (1986). Towards an articulatory phonology. *Phonology Yearbook, 3,* 219–252.

Browman, C., & Goldstein, L. (1992). Articulatory phonology: An overview. *Phonetica, 49,* 155–180.

Bryant, P., Bradley, L., MacLean, M., & Crossland, J. (1989). Nursery rhymes, phonological skills and reading. *Journal of Child Language, 16,* 407–428.

Bryant, P., MacLean, M., Bradley, L., & Crossland, J. (1990). Rhyme and alliteration, phoneme detection, and learning to read. *Developmental Psychology, 26,* 429–438.

Burgess, S. R., & Lonigan, C. J. (1998). Bidirectional relations of phonological sensitivity and prereading abilities: Evidence from a preschool sample. *Journal of Experimental Child Psychology, 70*(2), 117–141.

Buteau, C., & Hodson, B. (1989). *Phonological remediation targets: Words and primary pictures for highly unintelligible children.* Austin, TX: Pro-Ed.

Carlisle, J. (1995). Morphological awareness and early reading achievement. In L. Feldman (Ed.), *Morphological aspects of language processing* (pp. 189–209). Hillsdale, NJ: Erlbaum.

Carroll, J., & Snowling, M. (2004). Language and phonological skills in children at high risk of reading difficulties. *Journal of Child Psychology and Psychiatry, 45*(3), 631–645.

Carroll, J. M., Snowling, M. J., Hulme, C., & Stevenson, J. (2003). The development of phonological awareness in preschool children. *Developmental Psychology, 39*(5), 913–923.

Carrow-Woolfolk, E. (1999). *Test for Auditory Comprehension of Language* (3rd ed; TACL–3). Austin, TX: Pro-Ed.

Castle, J. M., Riach, J., & Nicholson, T. (1994). Getting off to a better start in reading and spelling: The effects of phonemic awareness instruction within a whole language program. *Journal of Educational Psychology, 86,* 350–359.

Castles, A., & Coltheart, M. (2004). Is there a causal link from phonological awareness to success in learning to read? *Cognition, 91*(1), 77–111.

Cataldo, S., & Ellis, N. (1988). Interactions in the development of spelling, reading and phonological skills. *Journal of Research in Reading, 11,* 86–109.

Catts, H., & Vartianen, T. (1993). *Sounds abound: Listening, rhyming and reading.* East Moline, IL: LinguiSystems.

Cheour, M., Ceponiene, R., Lehtokoski, A., Luuk, A., Allik, J., Alho, K., et al. (1998). Development of language-specific phoneme representations in the infant brain. *Nature Neuroscience, 1,* 351–353.

Cheung, H., Chen, H. C., Lai, C. Y., Wong, O. C., & Hills, M. (2001). The development of phonological awareness: Effects of spoken language experience and orthography. *Cognition, 81*(3), 227–241.

Chin, S., & Dinnsen, D. (1991). Feature geometry in disordered phonologies. *Clinical Linguistics and Phonetics, 5,* 329–337.

Chomsky, N., & Halle, M. (1968). *The sound pattern of English.* New York: Harper & Row.

Chugani, H. T. (1994). Development of regional brain glucose metabolism in relation to behavior and plasticity. In G. Dawson & K. W. Fischer (Eds.), *Human behavior and the developing brain* (pp. 153–175). New York: Guilford.

Churchill, J., Hodson, B., Jones, B., & Novak, R. (1988). Phonological systems of speech-disordered clients with positive/negative histories of otitis media. *Language, Speech, and Hearing Services in Schools, 19,* 100–107.

Clarke-Klein, S., & Hodson, B. (1995). A phonologically based analysis of misspellings by third graders with disordered-phonology histories. *Journal of Speech and Hearing Research, 38,* 839–849.

Clifton, L., & Elliott, L. (1982). CV identification thresholds for speech/language/learning-disordered listeners. *Journal of the Acoustical Society of America, 71,*

Compton, A. J. (1970). Generative studies of children's phonological disorders. *Journal of Speech and Hearing Disorders, 35,* 315–339.

Compton, A. J., & Hutton, J. S. (1978). *Compton-Hutton Phonological Assessment.* San Francisco: Carousel House.

Cossu, G., Shankweiler, D., Liberman, I., Katz, L., & Tola, G. (1988). Awareness of phonological segments and reading ability in Italian children. *Applied Psycholinguistics, 9,* 1–16.

Costello, J., & Onstine, J. M. (1976). The modification of multiple articulation errors based on distinctive feature theory. *Journal of Speech and Hearing Disorders, 41,* 199–215.

Cowan, W., & Moran, M. (1997). Phonological awareness skills of children with articulation disorders in kindergarten to third grade. *Journal of Children's Communication Development, 18*(2), 31–38.

Cupples, L., & Iacono, T. (2000). Phonological awareness and oral reading skill in children with Down syndrome. *Journal of Speech, Language, and Hearing Research, 43,* 595–608.

deBoysson-Bardies, B., Halle, P., Sagart, L., & Durand, C. (1989). A cross-linguistic investigation of vowel formants in babbling. *Journal of Child Language, 16,* 1–18.

Dean, E., & Howell, J. (1986). Developing linguistic awareness: A theoretically based approach to phonological disorders. *British Journal of Communication Disorders, 21,* 223–238.

Dean, E., Howell, J., Walters, D., & Reid, J. (1995). Metaphon: A metalinguistic approach to the treatment of phonological disorder in children. *Clinical Linguistics and Phonetics, 9*(1) 1–19.

Denton, C. A., Hasbrouck, J. E., Weaver, L. R., & Riccio, C. A. (2000). What do we know about phonological awareness in Spanish? *Reading Psychology, 21*(4), 335–352.

Dinnsen, D. A., Elbert, M., & Weismer, G. (1979, November). *On the characterization of functional misarticulations.* Paper presented at the annual convention of the American Speech-Language-Hearing Association, Atlanta, GA.

Dinnsen, D. A., Elbert, M., & Weismer, G. (1980, June). Some typological properties of functional misarticulation systems. In W. O. Dressler (Ed.), *Phonologica.* Paper presented at the Fourth International Phonology Meeting, Vienna, Austria.

Dodd, B. (1995). *Differential diagnosis and treatment of children with speech disorder.* London: Whurr.

Dodd, B., Crosbie, S., MacIntosh, B., Teitzel, T., & Ozanne, A. (2000). *Preschool and Primary Inventory of Phonological Awareness (PIPA).* London: Psychological Corporation.

Dodd, B., & Gillon, G. (2001). Exploring the relationship between phonological awareness, speech impairment and literacy. *Advances in Speech-Language Pathology, 3*(2), 139–147.

Dodd, B., Hua, Z., Crosbie, S., Holm, A., & Ozanne, A. (2003). *Diagnostic Evaluation of Articulation and Phonology.* London: Psychological Corporation.

Domnick, M., Coffman, G., Hodson, B., & Wynne, M. (1998, November). *Enhancing metaphonological skills of preliterate children with severe speech impairments.* Poster session presented at the annual convention of the American Speech-Language-Hearing Association, San Antonio, TX.

Donegan, P. J., & Stampe, D. (1979). The study of natural phonology. In D. A. Dinnsen (Ed.), *Current approaches to phonological theory* (pp. 126–173). Bloomington Indiana University Press, 126–173.

Duncan, L. G., & Johnston, R. S. (1999). How does phonological awareness relate to nonword reading skill among poor readers? *Reading and Writing, 11*(5–6), 405–439.

Dyson, A. T. (1988). Phonetic inventories of 2- and 3-year-old children. *Journal of Speech and Hearing Disorders, 53,* 89–93.

Dyson, A. T., & Paden, E. P. (1983). Some phonological acquisition strategies used by two-year-olds. *Journal of Childhood Communication Disorders, 7,* 6–18.

Edwards, H. T. (2003). *Applied phonetics: The sounds of American English* (3rd ed.). Clifton Park, NY: Delmar Learning.

Edwards, H. T., & Gregg, A. L. (2003). *Applied phonetics workbook: A systematic approach to phonetic transcription* (3rd ed.). Clifton Park, NY: Delmar Learning.

Edwards, M. L. (1979a). *Patterns and processes in fricative acquisition: Longitudinal evidence from six English-learning children.* Unpublished doctoral dissertation, Stanford University, CA.

Edwards, M. L. (1979b). Word position in fricative acquisition. *Papers and Reports on Child Language Development, 16,* 67–75.

Edwards, M. L. (1992). In support of phonological processes. *Language, Speech, and Hearing Services in Schools, 23,* 233–240.

Edwards, M. L. (1994). Phonological process analysis. In E. J. Williams & J. Langsam (Eds.), *Children's phonology disorders: Pathways and patterns.* Rockville, MD: American Speech-Language-Hearing Association.

Edwards, M. L., & Bernhardt, B. H. (1973a). *Phonological analyses of the speech of four children with language disorders.* Unpublished manuscript, Institute for Childhood Aphasia, Stanford University, CA.

Edwards, M. L., & Bernhardt, B. H. (1973b). *Twin speech as the sharing of a phonological system.* Unpublished manuscript, Institute for Childhood Aphasia, Stanford University, CA.

Edwards, M. L., & Shriberg, L. D. (1983). *Phonology: Applications in communicative disorders.* San Diego, CA: College-Hill Press.

Ehri, L. C., Nunes, S., Willows, D., Schuster, B., Yaghoub-Zadeh, Z., & Shanahan, T. (2001). Phonemic awareness instruction helps children learn to read: Evidence from the National Reading Panel's meta-analysis. *Reading Research Quarterly, 36*(3), 250–287.

Eilers, R. E. (1980). Infant speech perception: History and mystery. In G. Yeni-Komshian, J. Kavanagh, & C. A. Ferguson (Eds.), *Child phonology: Vol. 2. Perception* (pp. 23–39). New York: Academic Press.

Eimas, P., Siqueland, E., Jusczyk, P., & Vigorito, J. (1971). Speech perception in infants. *Science, 171,* 303–306.

Elbert, M. (1992). Consideration of error types: A response to Fey. *Language, Speech, and Hearing Services in Schools, 23,* 241–246.

Elbert, M., & Gierut, J. (1986). *Handbook of clinical phonology: Approaches to assessment and treatment.* San Diego, CA: College-Hill Press.

Elbro, C., Borstrom, I., & Petersen, D. K. (1998). Predicting dyslexia from kindergarten: The importance of distinctness of phonological representations of lexical items. *Reading Research Quarterly, 33*(1), 36–60.

Elliott, L., Longinetti, C., Clifton, L., & Meyer, D. (1981). Detection and identification thresholds for consonant-vowel syllables. *Perception and Psychophysics, 30,* 411–416.

Ezell, H. K., & Justice, L. M. (2000). Increasing the print focus of adult-child shared book reading through observational learning. *American Journal of Speech-Language Pathology, 9*(1), 36–47.

Fairbanks, G. (1954). Systematic research in experimental phonetics: A theory of the speech mechanism as a servosystem. *Journal of Speech and Hearing Disorders, 19,* 133–139.

Fairbanks, G. (1960). *Voice and articulation drillbook* (2nd ed.). New York: Harper Brothers.

Ferguson, C. A., & Farwell, C. B. (1975). Words and sounds in early language acquisition. *Language, 51,* 419–439.

Ferguson, C. A., & Garnica, O. K. (1975). Theories of phonological development. In E. Lenneberg & E. Lenneberg (Eds.), *Foundations of language development* (pp. 171–180). New York: Academic Press.

Ferguson, C. A., & Macken, M. A. (1980). Phonological development in children: Play and cognition. *Papers and Reports on Child Language Development, Stanford University, 18,* 133–177.

Fey, M. E. (1992). Clinical Forum: Phonological assessment and treatment articulation and phonology: An addendum. *Language, Speech, and Hearing Services in Schools, 23,* 277–282.

Fey, M. (2004, May). *EBP in child language intervention: Some background and some food for thought.* Paper presented at the conference of the Working Group on EBP in Child Language Disorders, Austin, TX.

Fey, M. E., & Gandour, J. (1982). Rule discovery in phonological acquisition. *Journal of Child Language, 9,* 71–81.

Flahive, L., Hodson, B., & Velleman, S. (2005, November). *Apraxia and Phonology.* Paper presented at the annual convention of the American Speech-Language-Hearing Association, San Diego, CA.

Flipsen, P., Jr., Hammer, J. B., & Yost, K. M. (2005). Measuring severity of involvement in speech delay: Segmental and whole-word measures. *American Journal of Speech-Language Pathology, 14*, 298–312.

Forrest, K. (2002). Are oral-motor exercises useful in the treatment of phonological/articulatory disorders? *Seminars in Speech and Language, 23*(1), 5–26.

Froehlich, D., Hodson, B., & Edwards, H. (2001). Characteristics of Vietnamese phonology: A tutorial. *American Journal of Speech-Language Pathology, 11,* 236–242.

Garrett, R. (1986). *A phonologically based speech improvement classroom program for hearing impaired students.* Unpublished manuscript, San Diego State University, San Diego, CA.

Gierut, J. (1989). Maximal opposition approach to phonological treatment. *Journal of Speech and Hearing Disorders, 54,* 9–19.

Gierut, J. (1990). Differential learning of phonological oppositions. *Journal of Speech and Hearing Research, 33,* 540–549.

Gierut, J. (1992). The conditions and course of clinically induced phonological change. *Journal of Speech and Hearing Research, 35,* 1049–1063.

Gierut, J. A. (2001). Complexity in phonological treatment. *Language, Speech, and Hearing Services in Schools, 32,* 229–241.

Gierut, J. A., Morrisette, M. L., Hughes, M. T., & Rowland, S. (1996). Phonological treatment efficacy and developmental norms. *Language, Speech, and Hearing Services in Schools, 27,* 215–230.

Gillon, G. (2000a). The efficacy of phonological awareness intervention for children with spoken language impairment. *Language, Speech, and Hearing Services in Schools, 31,*126–141.

Gillon, G. (2000b). *The Gillon phonological awareness training programme* (2nd ed.). Christchurch, New Zealand: University of Canterbury.

Gillon, G. (2000c). *Phonological awareness assessment materials for 3 and 4 year-old children.* www.cmds.canterbury.ac.nz/people/gillon.shtml

Gillon, G. (2002). Follow-up study investigating benefits of phonological awareness intervention for children with spoken language impairment. *International Journal of Language and Communication Disorders, 37*(4), 381–400.

Gillon, G. (2004). *Phonological awareness: From research to practice.* New York: Guilford Press.

Gillon, G. (2005). Facilitating phoneme awareness development in 3–4 year-old children with speech impairment. *Language, Speech, and Hearing Services in Schools, 36,*

Goldman, R., & Fristoe, M. (1969). *Goldman-Fristoe Test of Articulation.* Circle Pines, MN: American Guidance Service.

Goldman, R., & Fristoe, M. (2000). *Goldman-Fristoe Test of Articulations–2.* Circle Pines, MN: American Guidance Service.

Goldsworthy, C. (1998). *Sourcebook of phonological awareness activities: Children's classic literature.* San Diego, CA: Singular/Thomson Learning.

Good, R. H., & Kaminski, R. A. E. (2002). *Dynamic Indicators of Basic Early Literacy Skills (DIBELS;* 6th ed.). Eugene, OR: Institute for the Development of Educational Achievement.

Gordon-Brannan, M., & Hodson, B. (2000). Severity/Intelligibility measures of prekindergartners' speech. *American Journal of Speech-Language Pathology, 9,* 141–150.

Gordon-Brannan, M., Hodson, B., & Wynne, M. (1992). Remediating unintelligible utterances of a child with a mild hearing loss. *American Journal of Speech-Language Pathology, 1,* 28–38.

Grunwell, P. (1975). The phonological analysis of articulation disorders. *British Journal of Disorders of Communication, 10,* 31–42.

Grunwell, P. (1981). The development of phonology: A descriptive profile. *First Language, 3,* 161–191.

Grunwell, P. (1982). *Clinical phonology.* Rockville, MD: Aspen Systems Corporation.

Grunwell, P. (1985). *Phonological Assessment of Child Speech.* Windsor, England: NFER-Nelson.

Grunwell, P. (1987). *Clinical phonology* (2nd ed.). Baltimore: Williams & Wilkins.

Haelsig, P. C., & Madison, C. L. (1986). A study of phonological processes exhibited by 3-, 4-, and 5-year-old children. *Language, Speech, and Hearing Services in Schools, 17,* 95–106.

Harbers, H., Paden, E., & Halle, J. (1999). Phonological awareness and production: Changes during intervention. *Language, Speech, and Hearing Services in Schools, 30,* 50-60.

Hatcher, P. J. (1994). *Sound linkage: An integrated programme for overcoming reading difficulties.* London: Whurr.

Higgs, J. (1970). The articulation test as a linguistic technique. *Language and Speech, 13,* 262–270.

Higgs, J., & Hodson, B. (1978). Phonological perception of word-final obstruent cognates. *Journal of Phonetics, 6,* 25–35.

Hodson, B. (1975). *Aspects of phonological performance in four-year-olds.* Unpublished doctoral dissertation, University of Illinois.

Hodson, B. (1978). A preliminary hierarchical model for phonological remediation. *Language, Speech, and Hearing Services in Schools, 9,* 236–240.

Hodson, B. (1982). Remediation of speech patterns associated with low levels of phonological performance. In M. Crary (Ed.), *Phonological intervention: Concepts and procedures* (pp. 91–115). San Diego: College-Hill.

Hodson, B. (1983). A facilitative approach for remediation of a child's profoundly unintelligible phonological system. *Topics in Language Disorders, 3,* 24–34.

Hodson, B. (1986a) *Assessment of Phonological Processes–Revised.* Danville, IL: Interstate.

Hodson, B. (1986b). *Assessment of Phonological Processes–Spanish.* San Diego: Los Amigos.

Hodson, B. (1994a). Determining intervention priorities for preschoolers with disordered phonologies: Expediting intelligibility gains. *Children's phonology disorders: Pathways and patterns* (pp. 65–87). Rockville, MD: American Speech-Language-Hearing Association.

Hodson, B. (1994b). Helping individuals become intelligible, literate, and articulate: The role of phonology. *Topics in Language Disorders, 14,* 1–16.

Hodson, B. (1997). Disordered phonologies: What have we learned about assessment and treatment? In B. Hodson & M. Edwards (Eds.), *Perspectives in applied phonology* (pp. 197–224). Gaithersburg, MD: Aspen.

Hodson, B. (1998). Research and practice: Applied phonology. *Topics in Language Disorders, 18,* 58–70.

Hodson, B. (2001). Phonological cycles approach adapted for a child with a cochlear implant. *Proceedings of the International Association of Logopedics and Phoniatrics.* Montreal, Quebec.

Hodson, B. (2004). *Hodson Assessment of Phonological Patterns* (3rd ed.; HAPP–3). Austin, TX: Pro-Ed.

Hodson, B. (2003). Hodson Computerized Analysis of Phonological Patterns (HCAPP) [Computer software]. Wichita, KS: Phonocomp Software.

Hodson, B. (2005). *Enhancing phonological and metaphonological skills of children with highly unintelligible speech.* Rockville, MD: American Speech-Language-Hearing Association.

Hodson, B. W., & Paden, E. P. (1981). Phonological processes which characterize unintelligible and intelligible speech in early childhood. *Journal of Speech and Hearing Disorders, 46,* 369–373.

Hodson, B., & Paden, E. (1983). *Targeting intelligible speech: A phonological approach to remediation.* Austin, TX: Pro-Ed.

Hodson, B., & Paden, E. (1991). *Targeting intelligible speech: A phonological approach to remediation* (2nd ed.). Austin, TX: Pro-Ed.

Hodson, B., Buckendorf, R., Conrad, R., & Swanson, T. (1994). *Enhancing metaphonological skills of highly unintelligible 6-year-olds.* Poster presented at the annual convention of the American Speech-Language-Hearing Association, New Orleans, LA.

Hodson, B., Chin, L., Redmond, B., & Simpson, R. (1983). Phonological evaluation and remediation of speech deviations of a child with a repaired cleft palate: A case study. *Journal of Speech and Hearing Disorders, 48,* 93–98.

Hodson, B., Nonomura, C., & Zappia, M. (1989). Phonological disorders: Impact on academic performance? *Seminars in Speech and Language, 10,* 252–259.

Hodson, B., Scherz, J., & Strattman, K. (2002). Evaluating communicative abilities of a highly unintelligible child. *American Journal of Speech-Language Pathology, 11,* 236–242.

Hodson, B. W., & Strattman, K. H. (2004). Phonological awareness intervention for children with expressive phonological impairments. In R. Kent (Ed.), *MIT encyclopedia of communicative disorders* (pp. 153–156), Cambridge, MA: MIT Press.

Hoffman, P., Norris, J., & Monjure, J. (1990). Comparison of process targeting and whole language treatment for phonologically delayed preschool children. *Language, Speech, and Hearing Services in Schools, 21,* 102–109.

Holm, A., & Dodd, B. (1996). The effect of first written language on the acquisition of literacy. *Cognition, 59,* 119–147.

Howell, J., & Dean, E. (1994). *Treating phonological disorders in children* (2nd ed.). London: Whurr.

Hunt, J. (1961). *Intelligence and experience.* New York: Ronald Press.

Huttenlocher, P. R. (1994). Synaptogenesis in human cerebral cortex. In G. Dawson & K. W. Fischer (Eds.), *Human behavior and the developing brain* (pp. 35–54). New York: Guilford.

Ingram, D. (1974a). Fronting in child phonology. *Journal of Child Language, 1,* 233–241.

Ingram, D. (1974b). Phonological rules in young children. *Journal of Child Language, 1,* 49–64.

Ingram, D. (1976). *Phonological disability in children.* New York: Elsevier.

Ingram, D. (1983). Case studies of phonological disability. *Topics in Language Disorders, 3*(2),

Ingram, D. (1986). Explanation and phonological remediation. *Child Language Teaching and Therapy, 2,* 1–19.

Ingram, D., & Ingram, K. (2001). A whole-word approach to phonological analysis and intervention. *Language, Speech, and Hearing Services in Schools, 32,* 271–283.

International Phonetic Association. (2005). *International phonetic alphabet.* Retrieved 4/6/06 from http://www.arts.gla.ac.uk/ipa/images/pulmonic.gif

Invernizzi, M., Meier, J., & Juel, C. (2002). *Phonological Awareness Literacy Screening 1–3* (3rd ed.). Charlottesville, VA: University of Virginia Press.

Invernizzi, M., Meier, J., Swank, L., & Juel, C. (2002). *Phonological Awareness Literacy Screening for Kindergarten* (PALS–K). Charlottesville, VA: University of Virginia Press.

Invernizzi, M., Sullivan, A., & Meier, J. (2002). *Phonological Awareness Literacy Screening for Preschool (PALS–PreK).* Charlottesville, VA: University of Virginia Press.

Jakobson, R. (1949). On the identification of phonemic entities. *Recherches Structurales. Travaux du Cercle Linguistique de Prague, V,* 205–213.

Jakobson, R. (1968). *Child language, aphasia and phonological universals* (A. R. Keiler, Trans.). The Hague: Mouton. (From *Kindersprache, Aphasie und allgemeine Lautgesetze:* Uppsala. Original work published 1941)

Jakobson, R., Fant, G., & Halle, M. (1952). *Preliminaries to speech analysis: The distinctive features and their correlates* (Tech. Rep. No. 13, MIT Acoustics Laboratory) Cambridge, MA: MIT Press.

Jakobson, R., & Halle, M. (1956). *Fundamentals of language.* The Hague: Mouton.

Jenkins, R. (1988). *Multisyllabic word productions of normally developing 5-, 6-, and 7-year-olds.* Unpublished master's thesis, San Diego State University, San Diego, CA.

Johnson, J. (1996). *Metaphonological awareness treatment: Enhancing emergent literacy skills in "at risk" first graders.* Unpublished master's thesis, Wichita State University, Wichita, KS.

Johnston, R. S., Anderson, M., & Holligan, C. (1996). Knowledge of the alphabet and explicit awareness of phonemes in pre-readers: The nature of the relationship. *Reading and Writing, 8*(3), 217–234.

Justice, L. M., & Ezell, H. K. (2000). Enhancing children's print and word awareness through home-based parent intervention. *American Journal of Speech-Language Pathology, 9*(3), 257–269.

Justice, L. M., & Ezell, H. K. (2004). Print referencing: An emergent literacy enhancement strategy and its clinical applications. *Language, Speech, and Hearing Services in Schools, 35*(2), 185–193.

Kamhi, A. (2005). Summary, reflections, and future directions. In A. Kamhi & K. Pollock (Eds.), *Phonological disorders in children* (pp. 211–228). Baltimore: Brookes.

Kelman, M. E., & Edwards, M. L. (1994). *Phonogroup: A practical guide for enhancing phonological remediation.* Greenville, SC: Super Duper® Publications.

Kent, R. D. (1982). Contextual facilitation of correct sound production. *Language, Speech, and Hearing Services in Schools, 13,* 66–76.

Kent, R. D. (1984). The psychobiology of speech development: Co-emergence of language and a movement system. *American Journal of Physiology, 246,* 888–894.

Kent, R. D. (1997). Gestural phonology: Basic concepts and applications in speech-language pathology. In M. Ball & R. Kent (Eds.), *The new phonologies: Developments in clinical linguistics.* San Diego: Singular.

Kent, R. D. (2004). Normal aspects of articulation. In J. Bernthal & N. Bankson (Eds.), *Articulation and phonological disorders* (5th ed.; p. 162). Boston: Allyn & Bacon.

Kent, R. D., & Murray, A. (1982). Acoustic features of infant vocalic utterances at 3, 6, and 9 months. *Journal of the Acoustical Society of America, 72,* 353–365.

Khan, L. M. L., & Lewis, N. P. (2002). *Khan-Lewis Phonological Analysis (KLPA–2).* Circle Pines, MN: American Guidance Service.

Kiparsky, P., & Menn, L. (1977). On the acquisition of phonology. In J. Macnamara (Ed.), *Language learning and thought* (pp. 47–78). New York: Academic Press.

Klein, H. B. (1981). Productive strategies for the pronunciation of early polysyllabic lexical items. *Journal of Speech and Hearing Research, 24,* 389–405.

Kuhl, P. K. (1987). Perception of speech and sound in early infancy. In P. Salapatek & L. Cohen (Eds.), *Handbook of infant perception: Vol. 2. From perception to cognition* (pp. 275–382). New York: Academic Press.

Ladefoged, P. (2001). *Vowels and consonants. An introduction to the sounds of languages.* Malden, MA: Blackwell.

Larrivee, L., & Catts, H. (1999). Early reading achievement in children with expressive phonological disorders. *American Journal of Speech-Language Pathology, 8,* 137–148.

Lasky, R. E., Syrdal-Lasky, A., & Klein, R. E. (1975). VOT discrimination by four to six and a half month old infants from Spanish environments. *Journal of Experimental Child Psychology, 20,* 215–225.

Leitao, S., & Fletcher, J. (2004). Literacy outcomes for students with speech impairment: Long-term follow-up. *International Journal of Language & Communication Disorders, 39*(2), 245–256.

Leitao, S., Hogben, J., & Fletcher, J. (1997). Phonological processing skills in speech and language impaired children. *European Journal of Disorders of Communication, 32,* 73–93.

Leonard, L. B., Newhoff, M., & Mesalam, L. (1980). Individual differences in early child phonology. *Applied Psycholinguistics, 1,* 7–30.

Leonard, L., Schwartz, R., Swanson, L., & Frome-Loeb, D. (1987). Some conditions that promote unusual phonological behaviour in children. *Clinical Linguistics and Phonetics, 1,* 23–34.

Lewis, B. A., Freebairn, L. A., & Taylor, H. G. (2000). Follow-up of children with early expressive phonology disorders. *Journal of Learning Disabilities, 33,* 433–444.

Lindamood, P., & Lindamood, P. (2004). *Lindamood Auditory Conceptualization Test (LAC-3).* Austin, TX: Pro-Ed.

Lindamood, P., & Lindamood, P. (1998). *The Lindamood phoneme sequencing program for Reading, spelling, and speech: The LiPS program* (3rd ed.). Austin, TX: Pro-Ed.

LIPP: Logical International Phonetics Programs (Version 2.10) [Computer software]. (2001). Miami, FL: Intelligent Hearing Systems.

Locke, J. L. (1983). *Phonological acquisition and change.* New York: Academic Press.

Lof, G. (2003). Oral motor exercises and treatment outcomes. *Perspectives in language learning and education, 10,* 7–11

Long, S. H., Fey, M. E., & Channell, R. W. (2006). Computerized Profiling (Version 9.7.0) [Computer Software]. Milwaukee, WI: Marquette University.

Lonigan, C., Burgess, S., Anthony, J. L., & Barker, T. A. (1998). Development of phonological sensitivity in 2- to 5-year-old children. *Journal of Educational Psychology, 90*(2), 294–311.

Lorentz, J. P. (1974). A deviant phonological system of English. *Papers and Reports on Child Language Development, 8,* 55–64.

Love, E., & Reilly, S. (1995). *A sound way: Phonological awareness activities for early literacy.* Melbourne: Longman.

Lowe, R. (1995). *Assessment Link between Phonology and Articulation–Revised.* Mifflinville, PA: ALPHA Speech and Language Resources.

Lundberg, I., Olofsson, A., & Wall, S. (1980). Reading and spelling skills in the first few years predicted from phonemic awareness skills in kindergarten. *Scandinavian Journal of Psychology, 21,*159–173.

MacDonald, G. W., & Cornwall, A. (1995). The relationship between phonological awareness and reading and spelling achievement eleven years later. *Journal of Learning Disabilities, 28,* 523–527.

Macken, M. A. (1980). Aspects of the acquisition of stop systems: A cross-linguistic perspective. In G. Yeni-Komshian, J. F. Kavanagh, & C. A. Ferguson (Eds.), *Child Phonology: Vol. 1. Production* (pp. 143–168). New York: Academic Press.

Macken, M. A., & Ferguson, C. A, (1983). Cognitive aspects of phonological development: Model, evidence, and issues. In K. E. Nelson (Ed.), *Children's language* (Vol. 4; pp. 252–282). Hillsdale, NJ: Erlbaum.

Mann, D., & Hodson, B. (1994). Spanish-speaking children's phonologies: Assessment and remediation. *Seminars in Speech and Language, 15,* 137–148.

Mann, V. (1987). Phonological awareness: The role of reading experience. In P. Bertelson (Ed.), *The onset of literacy: Cognitive processes in reading acquisition* (pp. 65–91). Cambridge, MA: MIT Press.

Martin, D., Colesby, C., & Jhamat, K. (1997). Phonological awareness in Panjabi/English children with phonological difficulties. *Child Language Teaching and Therapy, 13(1),* 59–72.

Masterson, J. J., & Bernhardt, B. (2001). Computerized Articulation and Phonology Evaluation System (CAPES). San Antonio, TX: The Psychological Corporation.

Mattingly, I. G. (1972). Reading, the linguistic process, and linguistic awareness. In J. F. Kavanagh & I. G. Mattingly (Eds.), *Language by ear and by eye: The relationships between speech and reading* (pp. 133–147). Cambridge, MA: MIT Press.

McCabe, R. B., & Bradley, D. P. (1975). Systematic multiple phonemic approach to articulation therapy. *Acta Symbolica, 6*(1) 2–18.

McCarthy, J. J., & Prince, A. S. (1995). Faithfulness and reduplicative identity. In J. N. Beckman, L. W. Dickey, & S. Urbaczyk (Eds.), *University of Massachusetts Occasional Papers, 18* (pp. 249–384). Amherst, MA: Graduate Linguistic Student Association, University of Massachusetts.

McDonald, E. T. (1964). *Articulation testing and treatment: A sensory motor approach.* Pittsburgh, PA: Stanwix House.

McKinley, N. L., Schreiber, L. R., Sterling-Orth, A. J., & Tobalsky, S. A. (1999). *Silly sounds playground: Building children's phonological awareness.* Greenville, SC: Super Duper® Publications.

McLeod, S., van Doorn, J., & Reed, V. A. (2001). Normal acquisition of consonant clusters. *American Journal of Speech-Language Pathology, 10,* 99–110.

McReynolds, L. V., & Bennett, S. (1972). Distinctive feature generalization in articulation training. *Journal of Speech and Hearing Disorders, 37,* 462–470.

McReynolds, L. V., & Engmann, D. L. (1975). *Distinctive feature analysis of misarticulations.* Baltimore: University Park Press.

McReynolds, L. V., & Huston, K. (1971). A distinctive feature analysis of children's misarticulations. *Journal of Speech and Hearing Disorders, 36,* 156–166.

Menn, L. (1975). Evidence for an interactionist-discovery theory of child phonology. *Papers and Reports on Child Language Development, 12,* 169–177.

Menn, L. (1976). Evidence for an interactionist-discovery theory of child phonology. *Papers and Reports on Child Language Development,* 12, 169–177.

Menn, L. (1978). Phonological units in beginning speech. In A. Bell & J. B. Hooper (Eds.), *Syllables and segments* (pp. 157–171). North-Holland.

Menn, L. (1980). Phonological theory and child phonology. In G. Yeni-Komshian, J. F. Kavanagh, & C. A. Ferguson (Eds.), *Child phonology: Vol. 1. Production.* New York: Academic Press.

Menyuk, P. (1968). The role of distinctive features in children's acquisition of phonology. *Journal of Speech and Hearing Research, 11,* 138–146.

Metsala, J. L. (1999a). The development of phonemic awareness in reading-disabled children. *Applied Psycholinguistics, 20*(1), 149–158.

Metsala, J. L. (1999b). Young children's phonological awareness and nonword repetition as a function of vocabulary development. *Journal of Educational Psychology, 91*(1), 3–19.

Mody, M. (2003). Phonological basis in reading disability: A review and analysis of the evidence. *Reading and Writing: An Interdisciplinary Journal, 16,* 21–39.

Monnin, L. (1984). Speech sound discrimination testing and training: Why? Why not? In H. Winitz (Ed.), *Treating articulation disorders: For clinicians by clinicians* (pp. 1–20). Austin, TX: Pro-Ed.

Morris, S., Wilcox, K., Schooling, T. (1995). The Preschool/Speech Intelligibility Measure. *American Journal of Speech-Language Pathology, 4*(4), 22–28.

Montgomery, J., & Bonderman, R. (1989). Serving preschool children with severe phonological disorders. *Language, Speech, and Hearing Services in Schools, 20,* 76–83.

Mowrer, D. E. (1977). *Methods for modifying speech behaviors.* Columbus, OH: Merrill.

Mowrer, D. E. (1989). The behavioral approach to treatment. In N. Creaghead, P. Newman, & W. Secord (Eds.) *Assessment and remediation of articulatory and phonological disorders* (2nd ed.; pp. 159–192). Columbus, OH: Merrill.

Mowrer, D. E., Baker, R., & Schutz, R. (1968). *S-Programmed articulation control kit.* Tempe, AZ: Educational Psychological Research Associates.

Mowrer, O. H. (1952). Speech development in the young child: The autism theory of speech development and some clinical applications. *Journal of Speech and Hearing Disorders, 17,* 263–268.

Mowrer, O. H. (1960). *Learning theory and symbolic processes.* New York: Wiley & Sons.

Muter, V., Hulme, C., & Snowling, M. (1997). *Phonological Abilities Test (PAT).* London: Psychological Corporation.

Nathan, L., Stackhouse, J., Goulandris, N., & Snowling, M. (2004). The development of early literacy skills among children with speech difficulties: A test of the "critical age hypothesis." *Journal of Speech, Language, and Hearing Research, 47,* 377–391.

Newcomer, P., & Barenbaum, E. (2003). *Test of Phonological Awareness Skills (TOPAS).* Austin, TX: Pro-Ed.

Norris, J. A., & Hoffman, P. R. (1990). Language intervention within naturalistic environments. *Language, Speech, and Hearing Services in Schools, 21,* 72–84.

Northrup, P. (2002). *The literacy link.* Greenville, SC: Super Duper® Publications.

Notari-Syverson, A., O'Connor, R. E., & Vadasy, P. F. (1998). *Ladders to literacy: A preschool activity book.* Baltimore: Brookes.

Oller, D. K., (1973). Regularities in abnormal child phonology. *Journal of Speech and Hearing Disorders, 38,* 36–47.

Oller, D. K. (1980). The emergence of the sounds of speech in infancy. In G. Yeni-Komshian, J. Kavanagh, & C. A. Ferguson (Eds.), *Child phonology: Vol. 1. Production* (pp. 93–112). New York: Academic Press.

Olmsted, D. (1966). A theory of the child's learning of phonology. *Language, 42,* 531–535.

Olmsted, D. (1971). *Out of the mouth of babes.* The Hague: Mouton.

Paden, E. Pagel. (1970). *A history of the American Speech and Hearing Association 1925–1958.* Rockville, MD: American Speech and Hearing Association.

Paul, R. (2001). *Language disorders from infancy through adolescence: Assessment and intervention.* St. Louis, MO: Mosby.

Paget, R. (1963). *Human speech.* New York: Humanities.

Pollack, E., & Rees, N. (1972). Disorders of articulation: Some clinical applications of distinctive feature theory. *Journal of Speech and Hearing Disorders, 37,* 451–461.

Poole, E. (1934). Genetic development of articulation of consonant sounds in speech. *Elementary English Review, 11,* 159–161.

Porter, J. H., & Hodson, B. W. (2001). Collaborating to obtain phonological acquisition data for local schools. *Language, Speech, and Hearing Services in Schools, 32,* 165–171.

Prather, E., Hendrick, D., & Kern, C. (1975). Articulation development in children aged two to four years. *Journal of Speech and Hearing Disorders, 40,* 170–191.

Preisser, D. A., Hodson, B. W., & Paden, E. P. (1988). Developmental phonology: 18–29 months. *Journal of Speech and Hearing Disorders, 53,* 125–130.

Robb, M. P., & Bleile, K. M. (1994). Consonant inventories of young children from 8 to 25 months. *Clinical Linguistics & Phonetics, 8,* 295–320.

Robertson, C., & Salter, W. (1997). *The Phonological Awareness Test.* East Moline, IL: LinguiSystems.

Rosner, J. (1999). *Phonological awareness skills program.* Austin, TX: Pro-Ed.

Rosner, J. (1999). *Phonological Awareness Skills Test.* Austin, TX: Pro-Ed.

Rvachew, S., & Nowak, M. (2001). The effect of target-selection strategy on phonological learning. *Journal of Speech, Language and Hearing Research, 44,* 610–623.

Rvachew, S., Ohberg, A., Grawburg, M., & Heyding, J. (2003). Phonological awareness and phonemic perception in 4-year-old children with delayed expressive phonology skills. *Language, Speech, and Hearing Services in Schools, 12,* 463–471.

Sagey, E. (1986). *The representation of features and relations in non-linear phonology.* Unpublished doctoral dissertation, Massachusetts Institute of Technology, Cambridge, MA.

Sander, E. (1972). When are speech sounds learned? *Journal of Speech and Hearing Disorders, 37,* 55–63.

Scarborough, H. (1990). Very early language deficits in dyslexic children. *Child Development, 61,* 1728–1743.

Schmidt, L. S., Howard, B. H., & Schmidt, J. F. (1983). Conversational speech sampling in the assessment of articulation proficiency. *Language, Speech, and Hearing Services in Schools, 14,* 210–214.

Schreiber, L. R., Sterling-Orth, A. J., Thurs, S. A., & McKinley, N. L. (2000). *Working out with phonological awareness.* Greenville, SC: Super Duper® Publications.

Schwartz, R. (1992). Clinical applications of recent advances in phonological theory. *Language, Speech, and Hearing Services in Schools, 23,* 269–276.

Schwartz, R. G., & Leonard, L. B. (1982). Do children pick and choose? An examination of phonological selection and avoidance in early lexical acquisition. *Journal of Child Language, 9,* 319–336.

Scripture, M. K., & Jackson, E. (1927). *A manual of exercises for the correction of speech disorders.* Philadelphia, PA: F. A. Davis.

Secord, W., & Donahue, J. (2002). *Clinical Assessment of Articulation and Phonology (CAAP).* Greenville, SC: Super Duper.

Share, D., Jorm, A., MacLean, R., & Matthews, R. (1984). Sources of individual differences in reading acquisition. *Journal of Educational Psychology, 76,* 1309–1324.

Shields, M. (1997). *Enhancing metaphonological spelling skills of third graders with histories of phonological impairments.* Unpublished master's thesis, Wichita State University, KS.

Shine, R., & Proust, J. (1982). *Clinical treatment manual: Articulatory production training: A programmed sensory-motor approach.* Greenville, NC: East Carolina University.

Shriberg, L. (1997). Developmental phonological disorders: One or many? In B. Hodson & M. Edwards (Eds.), *Perspectives in applied phonology* (pp. 105–132). Gaithersburg, MD: Aspen

Shriberg, L. Allen, C., McSweeny, J. L., & Wilson, D. (2001). PEPPER: Programs to Examine Phonetic and Phonological Evaluation Records [Computer software]. Madison, WI: Waisman Center Research Computing Facility, University of Wisconsin-Madison.

Shriberg, L., Austin, D., Lewis, B., McSweeny, J., & Wilson, D. (1997). The percentage of consonants correct (PCC) metric: Extensions and reliability data. *Journal of Speech, Language, and Hearing Research, 40,* 708–722.

Shriberg, L. D., & Campbell, T. F. (Eds). (2002). *Proceedings of the 2002 childhood apraxia of speech research symposium.* Carlsbad, CA: The Hendrix Foundation.

Shriberg, L. D., & Kwiatkowski, J. (1980). *Natural process analysis (NPA): A procedure for phonological analysis of continuous speech samples.* New York: Wiley.

Shriberg, L., & Kwiatkowski, J. (1982). Phonological disorders III: A procedure for assessing severity of involvement. *Journal of Speech and Hearing Disorders, 47, 256–270.*

Singh, S., & Frank, D. C. (1972). A distinctive feature analysis of the consonantal substitution pattern. *Language and Speech, 15,* 209–218.

Small, L. H. (2005). *Fundamentals of phonetics: A practical guide for students* (2nd ed.). Boston: Pearson Education.

Smit, A. B. (1986). Ages of speech sound acquisition: Comparisons and critiques of several normative studies. *Language, Speech, and Hearing Services in Schools, 17,* 160–174.

Smit, A. B., & Hand, L. (1997). *Smit-Hand Articulation and Phonology Evaluation (SHAPE).* Los Angeles: Western Psychological Services.

Smit, A., Hand, L., Freilinger, J., Bernthal, J., & Bird, A. (1990). The Iowa articulation norms project and its Nebraska replication. *Journal of Speech and Hearing Disorders, 55,* 779–798.

Smith, M., Kneil, T., Hodson, B., Bernstorf, E., & Gladhart, M. (1994). *Rhyming abilities in children with impaired expressive phonologies.* Poster session presented at the annual convention of the American Speech-Language-Hearing Association, New Orleans, LA.

Smith-Kiewel, L., & Molenaar Claeys, T. (1998). *Once upon a sound.* Greenville, SC: Super Duper® Publications.

Snowling, M., Bishop, D. V. M., & Stothard, S. E. (2000). Is preschool language impairment a risk factor for dyslexia in adolescence? *Journal of Child Psychology and Psychiatry and Allied Disciplines, 41*(5), 587–600.

St. Louis, K., & Ruscello, D. (2000). *Oral Speech Mechanism Screening Examination* (3rd ed.) Austin, TX: Pro-Ed.

Stackhouse, J. (1992). Developmental verbal dyspraxia I: A review and critique. *European Journal of Disorders of Communication, 27,* 19-34.

Stackhouse, J. (1997). Phonological awareness: Connecting speech and literacy problems. In B. Hodson & M. Edwards (Eds.), *Perspectives in applied phonology* (pp. 157–196), Gaithersburg, MD: Aspen.

Stackhouse, J., & Wells, B. (1997). *Children's speech and literacy difficulties.* London: Whurr.

Stahl, S. A., & Murray, B. A. (1994). Defining phonological awareness and its relationship to early reading. *Journal of Educational Psychology, 86*(2), 221–234.

Stampe, D. (1969). The acquisition of phonetic representation. In R. T. Binnick, A. Davison, G. M. Green, & J. L. Morgan (Eds.), *Papers from the fifth regional meeting of the Chicago Linguistic Society* (pp. 443–454). Chicago, IL: Chicago Linguistic Society.

Stampe, D. (1972). *A dissertation on natural phonology.* Doctoral dissertation, University of Chicago, IL.

Stampe, D. (1973). *A dissertation on natural phonology.* Unpublished doctoral dissertation, University of Chicago. Revised version of 1972, *How I spent my summer vacation,* Ohio State University. (Also published as Stampe, D., 1979, *A dissertation on natural phonology.* New York: Garland Publishing.)

Stanovich, K. (1985). Explaining the variance in reading ability in terms of psychological processes. What have we learned? *Annals of Dyslexia, 35,* 67–96.

Stanovich, K. (1986). Matthew effects in reading: Some consequences of individual differences in the acquisition of literacy. *Reading Research Quarterly, 21,* 360–407.

Stark, R. E. (1980). Stages of speech development in the first year of life. In G. Yeni-Komshian, J. Kavanagh, and C. A. Ferguson (Eds.), *Child phonology: Vol. 1. Production* (pp. 73–92). New York: Academic Press.

Stemberger, J. P., & Bernhardt, B. H. (1997). Optimality theory. In M. J. Ball & R. D. Kent (Eds.), *The new phonologies: Developments in clinical linguistics.* San Diego: Singular Publishing Group.

Sterling-Orth, A. (2004). *Go-to guide for phonological awareness.* Greenville, SC: Super Duper® Publications.

Stinchfield, S. M., & Young, E. H. (1938). *Children with delayed or defective speech.* Stanford, CA: Stanford University Press.

Stoel-Gammon, C. (1985). Phonetic inventories, 15–24 months: A longitudinal study. *Journal of Speech and Hearing Research, 28,* 505–512.

Stoel-Gammon, C. (1992). Research on phonological development: Recent advances. In C. A. Ferguson, L. Menn, C. Stoel-Gammon (Eds.), *Phonological development: Models, research, implications* (pp. 273–281). Parkton, MD: York Press.

Stoel-Gammon, C., & Cooper, J. A. (1984). Patterns of early lexical and phonological development. *Journal of Child Language, 11,* 247–271.

Stoel-Gammon, C., & Dunn, C. (1985). *Normal and disordered phonology in children.* Austin, TX: Pro-Ed.

Stone, J. (1995). *Animated literacy.* La Mesa, CA: J. Stone Creations.

Streeter, L. A. (1976). Language perception of 2-month-old infants shows effects of both innate mechanisms and experience. *Nature, 259,* 39–41.

Stuart, M. (1995). Prediction and qualitative assessment of five- and six-year-old children's reading: A longitudinal study. *British Journal of Educational Psychology, 65,* 287–296.

Templin, M. (1957). *Certain language skills in children.* Minneapolis, MN: University of Minnesota Press.

Torgesen, J., & Bryant, B. (1994). *Test of Phonological Awareness.* Austin, TX: Pro-Ed.

Torgesen, J., Wagner, R., & Rashotte, C. (1994). Longitudinal studies of phonological processing and reading. *Journal of Learning Disabilities, 27,* 276–286.

Torgesen, J., Wagner, R., Rashotte, C., Lindamood, P., Rose, E., Conway, T., et al. (1999). Preventing reading failure in young children with phonological processing disabilities: Group and individual responses to instruction. *Journal of Educational Psychology, 91,* 579–593.

Trehub, S. E. (1976). The discrimination of foreign speech contrasts by infants and adults. *Child Development, 47,* 466–472.

Tunmer, W. E., Herriman, M. L., & Nesdale, A. R. (1988). Metalinguistic abilities and beginning reading. *Reading Research Quarterly, 23*(2), 134–158.

Tyler, A. A., Edwards, M. L., & Saxman, J. H. (1987). Clinical application of two phonologically based treatment procedures. *Journal of Speech and Hearing Disorders, 52,* 393–409.

Tyler, A. A., Lewis, K., Haskill, A., & Tolbert, L. (2002). Efficacy and cross domain effects of morphosyntax and a phonological intervention. *Language, Speech, & Hearing Services in Schools, 33,* 52–66.

Van Riper, C. (1934). *Speech correction: Principles and methods.* Englewood Cliffs, NJ: Prentice-Hall.

Van Riper, C. (1939). *Speech correction: Principles and methods* (2nd ed.). Englewood Cliffs, NJ: Prentice-Hall.

Van Riper, C. (1947). *Speech correction: Principles and methods* (3rd ed.). Englewood Cliffs, NJ: Prentice-Hall.

Van Riper, C. (1954). *Speech correction: Principles and methods* (4th ed.). Englewood Cliffs, NJ: Prentice-Hall.

Van Riper, C. (1963). *Speech correction: Principles and methods* (4th ed.). Englewood Cliffs, NJ: Prentice-Hall.

Van Riper, C. (1972). *Speech correction: Principles and methods* (5th ed.). Englewood Cliffs, NJ: Prentice-Hall.

Van Riper, C. (1978). *Speech correction: Principles and methods* (6th ed.). Englewood Cliffs, NJ: Prentice-Hall.

Van Riper, C. G., & Emerick, L. (1984). *Speech correction: An introduction to speech pathology and audiology* (7th ed.). Englewood Cliffs, NJ: Prentice-Hall.

Van Riper, C. G., & Erickson, R. (1996). *Speech correction: An introduction to speech pathology and audiology* (9th ed.). Englewood Cliffs, NJ: Prentice-Hall.

Velleman, S. (2002). Phonotactic therapy. *Seminars in Speech and Language, 23,* 43–56.

Velleman, S. (2003). *Childhood apraxia of speech resource guide.* Clifton Park, NY: Delmar Learning.

Velleman, S. (2005). Perspectives on assessment. In A. Kamhi & K. Pollock (Eds.), *Phonological disorders in children* (pp. 23–34). Baltimore: Brookes.

Velleman, S. L., & Shriberg, L. D. (1999). Metrical analysis of children with suspected developmental apraxia of speech. *Journal of Speech, Language, and Hearing Research, 42,* 1444–1460.

Vellutino, F., & Scanlon, D. (1987). Phonological coding, phonological awareness, and reading ability: Evidence from a longitudinal and experimental study. *Merrill-Palmer Quarterly, 33,* 321–363.

Vihman, M. M. (1976). From pre-speech to speech: On early phonology. *Papers and Reports on Child Language Development, 12,* 230–243.

Vihman, M. M. (1981). Phonology and the development of the lexicon: Evidence from children's errors. *Journal of Child Language, 8,* 239–264.

Vihman, M. M. (1998a). Early phonological development. In J. E. Bernthal & N. W. Bankson (Eds.), *Articulation and phonological disorders* (pp. 63–112). Needham Heights, MA: Allyn & Bacon.

Vihman, M. M. (1998b). Later phonological development. In J. E. Bernthal, & N. W. Bankson (Eds.), *Articulation and phonological disorders* (pp. 113–147). Needham Heights, MA: Allyn & Bacon.

Vihman, M. M., Ferguson, C. A., & Elbert, M. (1986). Phonological development from babbling to speech: Common tendencies and individual differences. *Applied Psycholinguistics, 7,* 3–40.

Vihman, M. M., & Greenlee, M. (1987). Individual differences in phonological development: Ages one to three years. *Journal of Speech and Hearing Research, 30,* 503–521.

Vygotsky, L. (1962). *Thought and language.* Cambridge, MA: MIT Press.

Vygotsky, L. (1978). *Mind in society: The development of higher psychological processes.* Cambridge, MA: Harvard Press.

Wagner, R., & Torgesen, J. (1987). The nature of phonological processing and its causal role in the acquisition of reading skills. *Psychological Bulletin, 101,* 192–212.

Wagner, R., Torgesen, J., & Rashotte, C. (1999). *Comprehensive Test of Phonological Processing (CTOPP).* Austin, TX: Pro-Ed.

Walley, A. C., Metsala, J. L., & Garlock, V. M. (2003). Spoken vocabulary growth: Its role in the development of phoneme awareness and early reading ability. *Reading and Writing: An Interdisciplinary Journal, 16,* 5–20.

Walsh, S. (2002). *Phonological awareness success.* Greenville, SC: Super Duper® Publications.

Waterson, N. (1970). Some speech forms of an English child: A phonological study. *Transactions of the Philological Society,* 1–24.

Waterson, N. (1971). Child phonology: A prosodic view. *Journal of Linguistics, 7,* 179–211.

Watson, M., & Lof, G. (2005). *Survey of universities' teaching: Oral motor exercises & other procedures.* Poster session presented at the annual convention of the American Speech-Language-Hearing Association, San Diego, CA.

Webster, P., & Plante, A. (1992). Effects of phonological impairment on word, syllable, and phoneme segmentation and reading. *Language, Speech, and Hearing Services in Schools, 23,* 176–182.

Webster, P., & Plante, A. (1995). Productive phonology and phonological awareness in preschool children. *Applied Psycholinguistics, 16* (1), 43–57.

Weiner, F. (1979). *Phonological Process Analysis.* Baltimore: University Park Press.

Weiner, F. (1981). Treatment of phonological disability using the method of meaningful minimal contrasts: Two case studies. *Journal of Speech and Hearing Disorders, 46,* 97–103.

Weismer, G., Tjaden, K., & Kent, R.D. (1995a). Can articulatory behavior in speech disorders be accounted for by theories of normal speech production? *Journal of Phonetics, 23,* 149–164.

Weismer, G., Tjaden, K., & Kent, R. D. (1995b). Speech production theory and articulatory behavior in motor speech disorders. In F. Bell-Berti & L. J. Raphael (Eds.), *Producing speech: Contemporary issues* (for Katherine Safford Harris; pp. 35–50). New York: American Institute of Physics.

Wellman, B. L., Case, I. M., Mengert, E. G., & Bradbury, D. E. (1931). Speech sounds of young children. *University of Iowa Studies in Child Welfare, 5,* 1–82.

Williams, A. L. (2000a). Multiple oppositions: Case studies of variables in phonological intervention. *American Journal of Speech-Language Pathology, 9,* 289–299.

Williams, A. L. (2000b). Multiple oppositions: Theoretical foundations for an alternative contrastive intervention approach. *American Journal of Speech-Language Pathology, 9,* 282–288.

Williams, P., & Stackhouse, J. (2000). Rate, accuracy and consistency: Diadochokinetic performance of young normally developing children. *Clinical Linguistics and Phonetics, 14,* 267-293.

Winitz, H. (1969). *Articulatory acquisition and behavior.* Englewood Cliffs, NJ: Prentice-Hall.

Winitz, H. (1975). *From syllable to conversation.* Baltimore: University Park Press.

Winitz, H., & Bellerose, B. (1962). Sound discrimination as a function of pretraining conditions. *Journal of Speech and Hearing Research, 5,* 340–348.

Author Index

Subject Index

Notes

Notes

Notes

About the Author

Barbara Williams Hodson, PhD, CCC-SLP, & Board Recognized Specialist in Child Language, is the author of English and Spanish phonological assessment instruments and the developer of a computer software program, the *Hodson Computerized Analysis of Phonological Patterns* (3rd ed.; 2003). Her other major publications include: *Targeting Intelligible Speech: A Phonological Approach to Remediation* (2nd ed.; 1991; with E. Paden); a *Topics in Language Disorders* theme issue, *From Phonology to Metaphonology* (1994), and *Perspectives in Applied Phonology* (1997, with M.L. Edwards). In addition, she has published a number of chapters in textbooks and numerous research articles in scholarly journals and has given several hundred Clinical Phonology presentations nationally and internationally. Prior to joining the faculty at Wichita State University, Hodson taught at San Diego State University and at the University of Illinois, the institution where she received her doctorate. She is a Fellow of the California and the American Speech-Language-Hearing Associations and was the recipient of the state Clinical Achievement Award for California in 1987 and for Kansas in 1992. Hodson, who has been directly involved in University Phonology clinics since 1975, received the 2004 American Speech-Language-Hearing Foundation's Frank R. Kleffner Lifetime Clinical Career Award.